# Lower Cholesterol And Triglycerides

## The Ultimate Guide To Optimal Health: Transforming Your Lifestyle For Longevity

Marta Sellers

*Lower Cholesterol And Triglycerides*

**Prose Books**
Prose Books LLC
Merrimack, NH 03054  USA
email: info@prosebooks.us

ISBN 978-1-963160-04-8

US$10.88

9 781963 160048

# Forward

In a world where health information is readily available but often contradictory, I am delighted to introduce *"Lowering Cholesterol and Triglycerides: The Ultimate Guide to Optimal Health Transforming Your Lifestyle for Longevity."* This book isn't a manual; it's a journey into the essence of what it means to live a balanced and healthy life.

Authored by Marta Sellers, a name with groundbreaking work in the field of holistic health, this book serves as a beacon of clarity and wisdom. Marta brings her expertise and profound understanding of the body to light as she addresses one of the most critical health concerns of our time: maintaining ideal cholesterol and triglyceride levels.

However, this book surpasses numbers and clinical recommendations. It delves into the equilibrium between physical well-being, mental wellness, and emotional harmony. Marta's approach doesn't rely on fixes or universal solutions; instead, it focuses on lifestyle transformations. She skillfully combines insights with everyday advice, making this book an invaluable resource for anyone seeking to enhance their overall health.

Each chapter is thoughtfully crafted with readers in mind, addressing questions and concerns with empathy and expertise. Marta takes the readers on a journey of health and wellness, covering topics like cholesterol, triglycerides, sleep, nutrition, and integrative health practices.

What makes this book unique is its focus on individuality. Marta acknowledges that each reader's path is different and encourages an approach to well-being. Her writing not only provides information but motivates and inspires positive changes for long-term health.

As you delve into these pages, you embark on a journey that goes beyond health measurements. Marta Sellers, your guide, understands that the ultimate goal is not about reducing cholesterol or triglycerides; it's about embracing vitality, longevity, and joy in life.

Welcome to your quest for well-being.

# Dedication

I want to express my gratitude to all those who find themselves at a crossroads seeking a path toward a more vibrant life.

To the individuals silently battling cholesterol and triglycerides whose struggles often remain unseen but deeply felt during moments of solitude. Your resilience and determination to carve out a better, healthier future serve as inspiration that lies within these pages.

To the families and friends who stand by and nurture those embarking on their health journeys. Your unwavering support and understanding form the foundation upon which transformations are built. You are the heroes in the story of being and recovery.

To the healthcare professionals, dietitians, fitness experts, and researchers committed to unraveling the complexities of health and wellness. Your tireless efforts in improving lives do not go unnoticed. This book serves as a testament to the knowledge and wisdom you generously share with the world.

Lastly, I extend my gratitude for my journey, which was filled with valuable lessons learned along the way, from nights spent researching and mornings devoted to writing to countless conversations that have shaped my understanding of health and well-being. This book is not a reflection of my experiences. Also encompasses shared experiences with many others.

May *"Lowering Cholesterol and Triglycerides: A Comprehensive Guide to Optimal Health Transforming Your Lifestyle for Longevity"* be a beacon of hope and a source of knowledge for everyone navigating the challenging realm of health and well-being.

May it motivate, enlighten, and lead you toward a life filled with equilibrium, good health, and longevity.

This extended dedication aims to acknowledge the range of individuals who contribute to and are impacted by the journey towards health. It is crafted to resonate with an audience, including those facing health challenges, their support networks, and professionals in the field.

## Table of Contents

# Chapter 1: Introduction

## Overview of the book's purpose and goals

Welcome to the journey towards achieving health! In this book, we embark on a quest to explore the importance of maintaining health and its profound impact on living a more fulfilling life. Through an examination of lifestyle choices, habits, and practices, our aim is to provide you with steps that can help improve your well-being and discover the secrets to leading a healthier life.

The purpose of this book is to shed light on the connection between our lifestyle choices and our overall health. By delving into the research incorporating holistic perspectives and drawing wisdom from ancient traditions, we strive to present a comprehensive approach to well-being. Our ultimate goal is to empower you as the reader to take control of your health by making decisions that will optimize your physical, mental, and emotional vitality.

## Understanding the significance of maintaining health and its impact on longevity

We currently live in a fast-paced era where busy schedules, sedentary lifestyles, and an abundance of processed foods have unfortunately become commonplace.

Consequently, poor health has become all too common for individuals. However, we all must recognize that our well-being serves as the foundation upon which our entire lives are built.

Without health, our ability to pursue our dreams, fulfill our responsibilities, and experience joy and happiness is compromised.

Maintaining health goes beyond preventing illness or managing symptoms. It's a continuous journey towards overall well-being. When we prioritize our health, we unlock the potential for more life. It's not uncommon for people who adopt habits and make positive lifestyle changes to feel energized, mentally focused, emotionally resilient, and overall vital.

Numerous scientific studies have clearly shown the link between lifestyle choices and lifespan. Engaging in activity, eating a nutritious diet, effectively managing stress, building strong social connections, and engaging in fulfilling activities all contribute to living longer. This book will delve deeper into these areas by providing you with knowledge and tools to make choices that promote health and longevity.

## How this guide can help readers transform their lifestyle for health

Embarking on a journey to transform your lifestyle for health can be both exciting and overwhelming. This guide aims to be your trusted companion throughout the process by supporting you every step of the way.

Whether you're starting from scratch or aiming to refine your existing routines, this book presents a roadmap for accomplishing your health objectives.

We've structured this guide to offer you an understanding of the factors that contribute to optimal health. Each chapter delves into aspects of lifestyle choices, habits, and practices, all of which play roles in transforming your well-being. From nutrition and exercise to stress management and sleep, we leave no stone unturned in our pursuit to uncover the secrets of life.

Throughout this book, we'll provide evidence-based suggestions, practical tips, and insights from experts to empower you to make changes. We acknowledge that everyone's journey is unique; therefore, we encourage you to tailor these recommendations according to your circumstances and preferences.

In addition to the elements, this guide also aims to foster a shift in mindset. We'll explore the power of thinking, the significance of self-compassion, and the value of adopting a growth mindset. By nurturing an approach towards health, our intention is to motivate you to create transformations that extend beyond physical well-being alone.

As we conclude, remember that the decisions you make today hold the potential to shape your future.

By taking the step on this journey towards improved well-being, you are making a valuable investment in yourself. Allow this guide to be your companion as it leads you towards health, a long and fulfilling life, and a sense of vitality and meaning. Are you prepared to embark on this empowering adventure? Let us get started.

# Chapter 2: Understanding Cholesterol and Triglycerides

## Introduction:

Cholesterol and triglycerides have received attention in the field of health. These substances are often discussed due to their connection to health conditions and cardiovascular diseases. This chapter aims to provide an understanding of cholesterol and triglycerides, including their roles in the body's different types and their impact on health. Additionally, we will explore the link between levels of cholesterol/triglycerides and various health conditions.

## Explanation of Cholesterol and Triglycerides

Cholesterol and triglycerides are compounds naturally found within our bodies. They fall under the category of lipids, which are essential for numerous bodily functions. Contrary to belief, cholesterol plays a role in hormone production, vitamin D synthesis, and aiding digestion through bile acid production. On the other hand, triglycerides serve as the storage form of energy-rich fat within our bodies.

## Different Types of Cholesterol and Triglycerides:

When discussing cholesterol, it is crucial to differentiate between its types. Low-density lipoprotein (LDL) cholesterol is commonly referred to as "cholesterol as it transports cholesterol from the liver to cells throughout the body. Excessive LDL cholesterol can accumulate in arteries, leading to atherosclerosis and an increased risk of heart disease.

High-density lipoprotein (HDL) cholesterol, which is commonly referred to as "cholesterol, aids in the removal of cholesterol from the bloodstream. This process helps to reduce the risk of heart disease.

Likewise, triglycerides can be classified based on their impact on our well-being. Normal levels of triglycerides are important for providing energy. High levels can contribute to the development of cardiovascular disease, pancreatitis, and other health complications.

## The Impact of Cholesterol and Triglycerides on Health

When LDL cholesterol levels are high, they tend to accumulate in the arteries and form plaques in blood vessels. This condition is known as atherosclerosis. It restricts blood flow, thereby increasing the risk of heart attacks or strokes. Conversely, HDL cholesterol plays a role by transporting cholesterol from arteries to the liver for disposal. It aids in preventing plaque formation. Thus, maintaining levels of HDL cholesterol is crucial for maintaining cardiovascular health.

Elevated triglyceride levels are often associated with eating habits, obesity, lack of activity, and excessive alcohol consumption. These factors can contribute to metabolic syndrome—a combination of conditions that heightens the risk for heart disease, stroke, and type 2 diabetes. Moreover, high triglyceride levels have been linked to the development of pancreatitis—an inflammation in the pancreas that can be life-threatening.

## The Link Between Elevated Cholesterol/Triglycerides and Various Health Issues

Having levels of cholesterol and triglycerides has been identified as a risk factor for multiple health problems. One of the notable is disease, which includes heart attacks, strokes, and peripheral artery disease. When plaque builds up in the arteries, it restricts blood flow, potentially leading to life-threatening consequences.

Furthermore, studies have shown an association between cholesterol and triglyceride levels and the likelihood of developing type 2 diabetes. Increased cholesterol and triglyceride levels can disrupt insulin function. Interfere with glucose metabolism, raising the chances of insulin resistance and subsequent diabetes.

It's essential to recognize that high cholesterol and triglycerides don't act alone. They often coexist with risk factors. These may include high blood pressure, smoking, obesity, and a sedentary lifestyle. When these factors come together, they create an environment for the development of health issues.

## Conclusion

In this section, we have explored the core concepts of cholesterol and triglycerides—their roles within the body—. Discussed their types.

We've also covered the implications of having levels of cholesterol and triglycerides on our health, specifically when it comes to how they affect health and the increased likelihood of developing conditions like metabolic syndrome and type 2 diabetes.

Individuals need to understand cholesterol and triglycerides so they can make informed choices about their diet, exercise routines, and overall lifestyle. By keeping cholesterol and triglyceride levels in check, people can significantly reduce their chances of developing health issues and enhance their well-being. In the sections, we'll explore strategies for managing and maintaining healthy levels of cholesterol and triglycerides.

# Chapter 3: Balanced Nutrition for Optimal Health

## Introduction

In today paced society, it has become increasingly vital to prioritize our health. A crucial aspect of achieving and maintaining health involves following a rounded diet. This section aims to emphasize the importance of having an intake to promote overall well-being. We will delve into the roles that macronutrients and micronutrients play in our bodies and offer practical suggestions for incorporating healthy food choices into our daily meals and snacks.

## The Significance of a Balanced Diet for Optimal Health

Maintaining health necessitates following a diet. Such a diet provides the nutrients and energy required for our bodies to function properly, ward off illnesses, and support growth and development. Failure to consume amounts of nutrients can lead to various health problems, including nutrient deficiencies, compromised immune function, and an increased risk of chronic diseases such as obesity, diabetes, and heart disease.

## Macronutrients Powering Our Bodys Functions

Macronutrients are the nutrients that our bodies require in quantities on a daily basis in order to sustain their functions efficiently. They encompass carbohydrates, proteins, and fats—each playing a role within our bodies.

Carbohydrates serve as the source of energy for our bodies. They are found in foods such as grains, fruits, and vegetables.

Our bodies break down carbohydrates into glucose, which acts as fuel for cells and powers functions. To ensure a release of energy and obtain fiber, vitamins, and minerals, it is advisable to opt for complex carbohydrates like whole grains.

Proteins are the building blocks that contribute to repairing and constructing tissues, producing enzymes and hormones to support a robust immune system. Good sources of protein encompass lean meats, fish, poultry, legumes, and dairy products. It is recommended to diversify protein sources to ensure an intake of amino acids.

Contrary to the belief that demonizes fats, they are actually crucial for health. Fats serve as energy sources and aid in absorbing soluble vitamins A, D, E, and K. Incorporating healthy fats from avocados, nuts, seeds, olive oil, and fatty fish is important while limiting saturated and trans fats that can increase the risk of heart disease.

## Micronutrients The Helpers

While macronutrients provide the energy requirements for our bodies' functioning, micronutrients such as vitamins and minerals play a vital role in maintaining optimal health, albeit in smaller quantities. Vitamins are substances that our bodies need in quantities to function properly. They have a role in generating energy, boosting our system, and maintaining the health of our skin, eyes, and bones. We can obtain vitamins by having a diet that includes fruits, vegetables, whole grains, and lean proteins. In situations or regions with sunlight exposure, some people may need to take supplements for specific vitamins like vitamin D.

On the other hand, minerals are essential elements that are not derived from living organisms but are necessary for various bodily functions. They contribute to the strength of our bones, nerve functioning, and hormone production. Examples of minerals include calcium, iron, magnesium, and zinc. To ensure a supply of minerals in our body, it is advisable to incorporate a variety of foods like dairy products, leafy greens, nuts, and legumes into our Diet.

## Here are some helpful tips for including food choices in your meals and snacks

**1. Prioritize whole foods:** Opt for foods like fruits and vegetables instead of processed or packaged options.

**2. Plan your meals ahead:** Take some time to plan your meals and snacks in advance.

**To maintain a well-rounded diet while avoiding unhealthy decisions, it is important to follow these guidelines:**

**1. Mindful portion control:** Be conscious of the sizes of your servings to prevent overeating. Using plates and listening to your body's hunger and fullness cues can help in this regard.

**2. Embrace a variety:** Ensure that your plate is filled with an array of fruits and vegetables. The different colors signify varying profiles, so incorporating produce will ensure you receive a wide range of essential nutrients.

**3. Stay hydrated:** Throughout the day, make sure to consume plenty of water. Opt for water, herbal tea, infused water, or sugary beverages for a health-conscious choice.

**4. Moderation is key:** It's perfectly fine to indulge in treats or indulgences; remember to do so in moderation. Enjoying your foods in portions can help strike a balance between pleasure and maintaining a healthy approach to eating.

In conclusion, maintaining a balanced diet serves as the foundation for health. By understanding the roles played by macronutrients and micronutrients and incorporating nutritious food choices into our daily meals and snacks, we can ensure that our bodies receive the necessary nutrients they need to thrive. Embrace the power of nutrition as you take steps toward becoming a happier version of yourself.

# Chapter 4: Regular Exercise for a Healthy Body

In today's fast-paced society, taking care of our bodies can sometimes feel like a battle. However, one of the ways to achieve and maintain overall well-being is through regular physical activity. In this chapter, we will explore the advantages of exercise on our health, delve into its effects on cholesterol and triglyceride levels, and provide useful tips for incorporating exercise into a busy lifestyle while overcoming common obstacles.

**Benefits of Regular Physical Activity on Overall Health and Well-being:**

Engaging in regular exercise has a profound impact on our overall health and well-being. It helps us maintain weight, lowers the risk of diseases, improves cardiovascular health, boosts mood and mental well-being, enhances sleep quality, and increases energy levels.

**Weight Management:** One of the benefits of regular physical activity is its contribution to weight management. Physical exercise assists in burning calories, increasing metabolism, and building muscle mass – all essential factors for maintaining weight. By including both exercises, such as walking, running, swimming, or cycling, and strength training exercises, like weightlifting or bodyweight exercises, in our routine, we can significantly enhance our ability to manage weight effectively.

Regular physical activity plays a role in reducing the risk of illnesses, including heart diseases, type 2 diabetes, certain cancers, and osteoporosis. By engaging in exercise, we can improve our health by lowering blood pressure, boosting levels of HDL (cholesterol and enhancing blood circulation. Additionally, exercise helps to increase insulin sensitivity, which is crucial for preventing and managing type 2 diabetes.

Participating in activity not only benefits our physical health but also positively impacts our mental well-being. Exercise triggers the release of endorphins, commonly known as "feel good" hormones that reduce stress, anxiety, and depression. It can also boost self-confidence, improve function, stimulate creativity, and provide an outlet for release.

## Different types of exercise have effects on cholesterol and triglyceride levels—both markers for cardiovascular health.

Aerobic exercises such as walking, jogging, swimming, and cycling have been proven to raise HDL (cholesterol levels. This increase aids in removing LDL (cholesterol, from the bloodstream.

## Regular aerobic exercise can also help reduce the risk of heart disease and stroke.

**Strength Training Exercises:** Incorporating resistance or weightlifting strength training exercises has been found to improve cholesterol profiles. They can increase levels of HDL cholesterol (the "kind) and decrease levels of LDL cholesterol (the "bad" kind). While strength training may not directly impact levels, it does contribute to body composition by increasing muscle mass and reducing body fat. This indirectly supports control over triglycerides.

**Flexibility and Balance Exercise**: Flexibility and balance exercises, like yoga or Pilates, may not directly affect cholesterol and triglyceride levels. However, they play a role in physical well-being by improving posture, preventing injuries, and enhancing overall mobility. These benefits indirectly support a lifestyle.

Tips for Incorporating Exercise into a Busy Lifestyle and Overcoming Common Barriers With Schedules and many responsibilities, it's possible to incorporate regular exercise into your routine and enjoy its benefits. Here are some practical tips to help you get started:

**1. Prioritize and Schedule:** Treat exercise as a part of your day that cannot be compromised. Schedule it in your calendar like any important appointment, and make sure you stick to it.

**2. Make it Enjoyable:** Choose activities that you genuinely enjoy doing, as this will increase your motivation to stick with them. Whether you're into dancing, playing sports, or venturing out into nature for a hike, it's important to find an activity that brings you joy while keeping you active.

**Start off small:** Gradually increase the duration and intensity of your workouts over time. This approach ensures that you can sustain your exercise routine and reduces the risk of injury.

**Take advantage of breaks during work:** When doing household chores, squeeze in some physical activity. You can go for walks, do stretches, or even perform bodyweight exercises to keep yourself moving.

Getting friends or family involved in activities not only helps with accountability but also makes exercising more enjoyable. Consider joining group classes and organizing activities as a team.

Identify and address common obstacles that may hinder your exercise routine, such as lack of time, fatigue, or feeling self-conscious. Find solutions like waking up a bit, exploring exercise options, or incorporating physical activity into your daily routines, like walking or cycling to work.

In conclusion, regular exercise plays a role in maintaining a body and overall well-being. By understanding the effects it has on cholesterol and triglyceride levels and implementing strategies to overcome common barriers, we can prioritize physical activity and witness its transformative power firsthand.

Begin your journey today. Experience the long-term benefits of a more joyful life.

# Chapter 5: Stress Management Techniques

S tress has become a part of our lives, impacting both our physical and mental well-being. In this chapter, we will explore how stress affects our health and its connection to cholesterol and triglyceride levels. We will also delve into techniques for managing stress that can help alleviate its effects. By incorporating these techniques into our routines, we can reduce stress. Enhance our overall well-being.

## Understanding the Impact of Stress on Health and Cholesterol/Triglyceride Levels

Stress is not a matter of emotions; it deeply influences our health as well. When we experience stress, our bodies release cortisol, a hormone that prepares us for the fight or flight response. However, chronic stress can disrupt the balance within our bodies, leading to health issues, including problems related to cardiovascular health.

One significant connection between stress and health lies in their impact on cholesterol and triglyceride levels. High levels of stress can raise LDL cholesterol (commonly known as "cholesterol) and triglycerides while simultaneously reducing HDL cholesterol (known as "cholesterol). This combination increases the risk of heart disease and other complications related to health.

---

*The body's reaction to stress triggers a series of events that contribute to a profile of cholesterol levels.*

---

Stress has a tendency to trigger the release of fatty acids, which leads to levels of triglycerides. When triglyceride levels become excessive, it can result in the buildup of LDL cholesterol within artery walls, which increases the risk of atherosclerosis and heart disease. Additionally, stress can indirectly affect cholesterol by influencing our behaviors, such as overeating, consuming foods, or neglecting exercise.

## Various Techniques for Managing Stress

Thankfully, there are techniques available for managing stress and mitigating its negative impact on our health. Let us explore some of these techniques.

**Practicing Mindfulness:** Mindfulness involves being fully present in the moment and attentively observing our thoughts, emotions, and sensations without judgment. By practicing mindfulness through activities like meditation or deep breathing exercises or simply engaging in activities that bring us joy and fulfillment, we can detach ourselves from our thoughts and gain a clearer perspective on what causes us stress.

**Engaging in Meditation:** Meditation is a tool for reducing stress and promoting relaxation. By directing our focus and quieting our minds through meditation practices, we can calm down our system. Trigger the relaxation response. Consistent meditation practice has been proven to lower cortisol levels, decrease blood pressure levels, and enhance well-being. Starting a meditation routine doesn't have to be complicated; even dedicating a few minutes daily to meditation can yield benefits.

**Relaxation Techniques:** Engaging in relaxation techniques, like muscle relaxation or guided imagery, can bring relief from mental tension. Progressive muscle relaxation involves tensing and then releasing muscle groups to let go of accumulated stress. Guided imagery employs visualization methods to create calming images that transport us to a place of tranquility.

## Strategies for Reducing Stress and Enhancing Overall Well-being in Everyday Life

While it's crucial to incorporate stress management techniques into our routines, it's equally important to adopt strategies that minimize stress in our day-to-day lives. Here are some practical approaches worth considering

**Prioritize Self-Care:** Take time each day to engage in activities that promote self-care and relaxation. This can include exercising, pursuing hobbies, spending time with loved ones, or taking breaks for rejuvenation purposes. By prioritizing self-care, we strengthen our ability to handle stress and foster overall well-being.

**Set Realistic Goals:**  Establishing goals can create pressure and elevate stress levels. Instead, set objectives. Break them down into manageable steps. Celebrating victories along the way can provide a sense of accomplishment while reducing stress.

**Practice Effective Time Management:** Poor time management often leads to stress and feelings of being overwhelmed. Make sure to prioritize your tasks, delegate whenever possible, and create a schedule that allows for breaks and relaxation. By managing our time, we can reduce stress. Increase productivity.

It's important to surround ourselves with positive individuals as they can have an impact on our stress levels. Seek out friends, family members, or support groups who provide a space for sharing concerns and finding comfort. Social connections can offer perspectives and emotional support during times.

To wrap up this chapter, we delved into the effects of stress on our health and its connection to cholesterol and triglyceride levels. We also explored techniques for managing stress, such as practicing mindfulness, meditation, and relaxation exercises.

Lastly, we discussed strategies for reducing stress in our lives and improving well being. By incorporating these techniques and strategies into our lives, we can effectively manage stress while safeguarding our mental health. Remember that the journey towards stress management is ongoing; with determination and persistence, we can cultivate a more balanced life.

# Chapter 6: Disease Prevention and Your Health

Understanding the impact of cholesterol and triglyceride levels on our health is crucial, as they can lead to diseases and health conditions. This chapter aims to explore the consequences of these abnormalities and discuss ways to prevent them through lifestyle modifications and medical interventions. Additionally, we will emphasize the significance of health checkups and screenings for detection and prevention.

Cholesterol and triglycerides are lipids in our bodies. However, when their levels become excessively high, they can have effects on our health. High cholesterol levels increase the risk of atherosclerosis, a condition where fatty plaques accumulate in the arteries. These plaques cause narrowing and hardening of the arteries, which reduces blood flow and potentially leads to heart attacks and strokes. On the other hand, elevated triglyceride levels are associated with an increased risk of metabolic syndrome type 2 diabetes and pancreatitis.

## Lifestyle changes and interventions play a role in preventing these conditions.

Healthy Diet Adopting a diet that's low in saturated fats and trans fats while being rich in fruits, vegetables, whole grains, and lean proteins can effectively lower cholesterol and triglyceride levels.

To improve your profile and reduce the risk of diseases, it is important to make certain lifestyle changes. Firstly, avoid processed foods and excessive consumption of beverages. These can contribute to lipid abnormalities. Additionally, engaging in activities like brisk walking, jogging, cycling, or swimming can help lower cholesterol and triglyceride levels while improving heart health and maintaining a healthy weight.

Managing your weight through a diet and exercise is crucial in preventing cholesterol and triglycerides. Losing weight can significantly improve your profile and reduce the risk of complications associated with high levels. Lastly, quitting smoking is essential for health as it damages blood vessels, reduces cholesterol levels, and increases the risk of heart disease.

In some cases where lifestyle changes alone may not be enough to control cholesterol and triglyceride levels, medical interventions are necessary. Medications such as statins and fibrates may be prescribed by healthcare professionals to help manage these abnormalities by reducing cholesterol synthesis or increasing its elimination from the body.

Omega 3 fatty acids found in fish like salmon, mackerel, and sardines, as well as plant sources such as flaxseeds and walnuts, have also been proven effective in lowering triglyceride levels.

Omega 3 supplements might be suggested by healthcare professionals to complement lifestyle adjustments and medication therapy. The significance of health checkups and screenings for detecting and preventing diseases early.

Regular health checkups and screenings play a role in identifying and preventing diseases linked to levels of cholesterol and triglycerides. These screenings often involve blood tests to measure cholesterol levels as well as other important markers like blood pressure and blood glucose levels.

Detecting issues early enables healthcare professionals to intervene promptly, providing treatments and lifestyle modifications to halt the progression of these abnormalities and associated diseases.

Furthermore, health checkups provide an opportunity for healthcare providers to educate individuals about the importance of making lifestyle changes and the potential risks tied to cholesterol and triglycerides. They can offer personalized guidance on adjustments to exercise routines and stress management techniques aimed at optimizing health.

## Conclusion

In this section, we have explored an overview of ailments and health conditions associated with cholesterol and triglycerides. We have discussed methods for preventing these conditions through lifestyle changes and medical interventions. Lastly, we have emphasized the significance of health checkups and screenings in detecting issues for prevention purposes.

By taking a stance and making changes to our lifestyle, we can greatly decrease the likelihood of developing such ailments and enhance our general health and well-being.

# Chapter 7: Implementing Lifestyle Changes for Long-Term Success

C hapter 7 is dedicated to exploring the side of making lifestyle changes that lead to long-term success. We all know that altering our habits and embracing a lifestyle can be difficult. With the right guidance and motivation, it is entirely possible. This chapter aims to equip you with the tools, strategies, and tips for setting goals, designing a personalized health plan, overcoming challenges, and maintaining healthy habits in the long run.

When it comes to implementing lifestyle changes, it's crucial to set attainable goals. Unrealistic expectations can often result in disappointment and frustration, ultimately impeding our path toward health. Here are some steps you can follow to establish goals and create a health plan

**1. Assess Your Current Health Status:** Begin by evaluating your habits – both negative – across various aspects such as physical well-being, mental state, diet choices, exercise routines, and stress levels.

**2. Prioritize Areas for Improvement:** Once you have identified the areas you wish to transform or improve upon, prioritize them based on their significance to you as well as your overall health. Focusing on one or two areas at a time can help prevent overwhelm while increasing your likelihood of success.

**Here are some tips to help you set goals and stay motivated on your journey towards health:**

**1. Be Specific:** Make sure your goals are clear and well-defined. For a goal like "exercise more," set a specific goal like "I will exercise for 30 minutes, five days a week for the next three months."

**2. Break It Down:** Divide your goals into steps. This approach makes them more manageable. Keeps you motivated. For example, if you want to improve your diet, start by adding fruits and vegetables to your meals.

**3. Customize Your Health Plan:** Create a plan that includes your goals, the steps you'll take to achieve them, and a timeline for each milestone. Consider areas like exercise, nutrition, stress management, or any others that are important to you. Remember to remain flexible and adjust the plan as needed along the way.

**4. Overcoming Challenges:** Understand that implementing lifestyle changes can be difficult at times. It is not impossible! Stay and adopt strategies that work for you. With determination and perseverance, obstacles can be overcome.

**5. Staying Motivated:** Keep yourself motivated throughout the process by finding what inspires you personally. Whether it's tracking progress or rewarding yourself for reaching milestones. Find ways to celebrate victories along the way.

---

*Remember that achieving health is a journey rather than an overnight success story; embrace it with patience and commitment.*

---

**Here are some helpful suggestions to consider:**

**1. Seek Support:** It's important to have a network of people who share your goals or can provide guidance and motivation. You can join a support group, find a workout buddy, or even seek assistance if necessary.

**2. Embrace Gradual Change:** Try to embrace gradual change instead of making drastic changes overnight. Try incorporating new habits into your routine gradually. This approach allows for a transition. Increases the likelihood of long-term success.

**3. Celebrate Small Achievements:** Take the time to acknowledge and celebrate each milestone along your journey, no matter how small they may seem. Recognizing these accomplishments reinforces behavior. Keeps you motivated to continue.

**4. Learn from Challenges:** Accept that setbacks are a part of the process and view them as opportunities for growth. When faced with a setback, take the time to understand what factors contributed to it, learn from the experience, and make any adjustments moving forward.

**5. Practice Self-Compassion:** Be kind to yourself throughout this journey of change. Understand that it takes time, and setbacks do not define your success or failure. Treat yourself with compassion. Prioritize self-care in order to maintain a positive mindset.

## Strategies for Sustaining Healthy Habits and Making Long-Term Lifestyle Changes

Remember that creating habits is the beginning; sustaining them over the long term is what truly leads to lasting success.

Here are some tips to help you maintain habits and sustain your lifestyle changes

**1. Find Enjoyment:** Discover activities or healthy foods that genuinely bring you joy. If exercise feels like a chore, try activities until you find something that you truly enjoy. The more enjoyable it is, the more likely you'll stick with it.

**2. Practice Mindfulness:** Cultivate awareness of your habits, triggers, and emotions. Being mindful helps you make choices and avoid falling into old patterns. Take time to reflect on your progress regularly.

**3. Track Your Progress:** Keep a journal. Use technology to keep track of how you've come. Documenting your accomplishments, challenges, and emotions can provide insights. Keep you motivated.

**4. Adjust and Adapt:** As you progress on your journey, be open to adjusting your goals and strategies according to your changing needs and circumstances.

**5. Celebrate Milestones:** Embrace and celebrate your milestones along the way and celebrate when you achieve them! Reward yourself with food-related treats, like a massage or new workout gear, as a way to acknowledge your accomplishments.

## In conclusion

Chapter 7 offers guidance on setting goals, creating a health plan, overcoming challenges, and maintaining healthy habits.

Keep in mind that making lifestyle adjustments requires patience, dedication, and a commitment to consistency. If you adhere to these principles and stay focused, you'll be able to attain success on your path toward well-being.

# Chapter 8: Resources and Additional Support

When it comes to achieving health, it's important to understand that the journey should not be undertaken alone. Seeking support from resources can offer guidance, knowledge, and motivation. This chapter explores the range of resources and additional support available to individuals who are striving to improve their well-being.

From suggested reading materials, websites, and online resources to the significance of support groups, healthcare professionals, and community programs – this chapter provides an overview for those looking to enhance their wellness.

### Suggestions for Reading

Reading not only expands our knowledge but also serves as a powerful tool for personal growth and transformation. The following books are highly recommended for individuals seeking to deepen their understanding of health and well-being.

1. *"The Power of Now"* by Eckhart Tolle This transformative book delves into the significance of living in the moment and its positive impact on well-being.

2. *"The Blue Zones Lessons for Living from the People Who've Lived the Longest"* by Dan Buettner This captivating book examines the lifestyles and habits

of populations known for their longevity, offering insights into health and longevity.

3. *"The Wellness Revolution"* by Paul Zane Pilzer This book presents a perspective on the wellness industry. Delves into the economic implications of prioritizing health and well-being.

## Online Resources

The internet has completely transformed how we access information, making it incredibly convenient to find resources that support our quest for health. Here are some recommended websites and online resources

Mayo Clinic (www.mayoclinic.org) A trusted source for information, this website provides comprehensive resources covering various health conditions, treatments, and preventive measures.

National Institutes of Health (www.nih.gov) As a leading research institution, the National Institutes of Health offers a wealth of information and resources on health and wellness.

WebMD (www.webmd.com) With its collection of articles, expert opinions, and interactive tools, WebMD serves as a resource for understanding health conditions and adopting healthy lifestyle practices.

## Introduction to Support Groups, Health Professionals, and Community Programs

While books and online resources can offer insights, achieving health often requires the support and guidance of others. Support groups, health professionals, and community programs play roles in facilitating growth and well-being. Support

Groups Support groups provide a space where people who share experiences or challenges can come together.

These groups offer a sense of community, encouragement, empathy, and an opportunity to learn from others who have gone through situations. Whether it is a support group for weight loss, addiction recovery, or a specific health condition, they can be found at community centers, hospitals, or online platforms like Meetup.com and condition-specific forums.

Health Professionals It is crucial to seek guidance from healthcare professionals when dealing with health issues. Consulting with doctors, nurses, dietitians, and therapists can provide advice, treatment plans, and ongoing support. These professionals possess the expertise and experience needed to address needs and help develop strategies for achieving health.

Community Programs Communities often offer programs and initiatives aimed at improving the well-being of residents. These programs may include fitness classes, health screenings, support groups, and educational workshops. Community centers, religious organizations, and local government websites are resources for discovering and actively participating in these initiatives.

*On the journey towards health, it is important to understand that seeking guidance and support is nothing to be ashamed of.*

## Encouragement to Seek Additional Guidance and Support

In reality, receiving support can have an impact and help individuals overcome challenges to achieve their health goals more effectively. By connecting with support groups, healthcare professionals, and community programs, individuals can access a network of resources, knowledge, and encouragement that will propel them toward well-being.

## In conclusion

Chapter 8 has emphasized the range of resources and additional assistance to individuals who are striving to improve their health and well-being. By delving into recommended readings, exploring websites and online resources, engaging with support groups, consulting healthcare professionals, and participating in community programs, individuals can make progress toward achieving optimal health. It's essential to remember that the journey toward wellness should not be undertaken alone; seeking guidance and support can lead to transformative outcomes in attaining lasting well-being.

# Chapter 9: Frequently Asked Questions and Answers

**Questions and Answers:**

1. Q: What are the main types of cholesterol?

   A: The main types of cholesterol are Low-Density Lipoprotein (LDL), often referred to as 'bad' cholesterol, and High-Density Lipoprotein (HDL), known as 'good' cholesterol.

2. Q: Why is high LDL cholesterol harmful?

   A: High LDL cholesterol can build up in the walls of your arteries, leading to atherosclerosis, which increases the risk of heart attack and stroke.

3. Q: Can Diet affect cholesterol levels?

   A: Yes, Diet plays a significant role in cholesterol levels. Foods high in saturated and trans fats can increase LDL cholesterol, while foods rich in fiber and healthy fats can lower it.

4. Q: What is the role of fiber in cholesterol management?

   A: Dietary fiber, especially soluble fiber, helps reduce the absorption of cholesterol into the bloodstream.

5. Q: How does exercise influence cholesterol levels?

A: Regular exercise can help lower LDL cholesterol and raise HDL cholesterol, improving overall heart health.

6. Q: What are triglycerides, and why are they important?

A: Triglycerides are a type of fat found in the blood. High levels can increase the risk of heart disease, especially when combined with high LDL cholesterol or low HDL cholesterol.

7. Q: How does stress affect cholesterol levels?

A: Chronic stress can lead to unhealthy lifestyle choices and hormonal changes that may raise LDL and lower HDL cholesterol levels.

8. Q: What is the impact of sleep on cholesterol?

A: Poor sleep patterns have been linked to higher levels of LDL cholesterol and lower levels of HDL cholesterol.

9. Q: Can herbal remedies be used to manage cholesterol?

A: Certain herbal remedies may support cholesterol management, but they should be used under medical supervision as part of a comprehensive treatment plan.

10. Q: Is it necessary to eliminate all fats from the Diet to lower cholesterol?

A: No, it's important to choose healthy fats, such as those found in nuts, seeds, and fish, while limiting saturated and trans fats.

11. Q: Can losing weight help lower cholesterol levels?

A: Yes, weight loss, especially when coupled with a healthy diet and exercise, can help lower cholesterol levels.

12. Q: Are there specific foods that help lower cholesterol?

A: Foods like oats, nuts, fatty fish, olive oil, and fruits rich in fiber can help lower cholesterol.

13. Q: What is mindful eating, and how does it help?

A: Mindful eating is the practice of being fully present and aware during eating. It helps in better digestion, enjoying meals more, and can prevent overeating.

14. Q: How does gut health affect overall health?

A: A healthy gut contributes to a strong immune system, effective digestion, improved mood and sleep, and overall health, including heart health.

15. Q: What are the benefits of yoga for heart health?

A: Yoga can reduce stress, lower blood pressure, and improve circulation, all of which are beneficial for heart health.

16. Q: Why is it important to have regular health check-ups?

A: Regular health check-ups can help detect high cholesterol and triglycerides early, allowing for timely intervention.

17. Q: Can smoking affect cholesterol levels?

A: Yes, smoking can lower HDL (good) cholesterol and is a risk factor for heart disease.

18. Q: What role do antioxidants play in heart health?

A: Antioxidants help combat oxidative stress and inflammation, reducing the risk of heart disease.

19. Q: How important is it to tailor an exercise plan to individual needs?

A: Tailoring an exercise plan to individual needs ensures it is safe, effective, and sustainable, considering personal health conditions and fitness levels.

20. Q: What is the significance of setting achievable health goals?

A: Setting achievable health goals is important for motivation and progress. It helps in maintaining focus and measuring success in the journey towards better health.

These questions and answers cover key aspects of the book's content, providing readers with a concise overview and deeper understanding of the topics discussed.

# Chapter 10: Breakfast Recipes

Welcome to the Breakfast Recipe Section of "Lower Cholesterol And Triglycerides: The Ultimate Guide to Optimal Health: Transforming Your Lifestyle for Longevity." In this section, we will guide you through a collection of delicious and heart-healthy breakfast recipes specially crafted to help lower cholesterol and triglyceride levels. Breakfast is often considered the most important meal of the day, and making nutritious choices in the morning can set the tone for the rest of your day and your overall health journey.

**About the Book:**

"Lower Cholesterol And Triglycerides: The Ultimate Guide to Optimal Health" is your comprehensive resource for achieving and maintaining a heart-healthy lifestyle. This book is designed to empower you with knowledge and practical strategies to improve your cardiovascular health, reduce cholesterol and triglyceride levels, and increase your overall well-being. The breakfast recipes featured here are just one part of our holistic approach to better heart health.

**Why Focus on Breakfast?**

Starting your day with a wholesome, cholesterol-friendly breakfast can significantly impact your cholesterol and triglyceride levels. These recipes are tailored to provide essential nutrients, fiber, and healthy fats while avoiding excessive saturated and trans fats, which are known to raise cholesterol levels. Whether you're new to a heart-healthy diet or looking to expand your repertoire of breakfast options, these recipes are sure to please your taste buds while supporting your health goals.

**What to Expect:**

In this Breakfast Recipe Section, you'll find a diverse range of breakfast ideas, from hearty classics to creative and unique dishes. Our recipes are designed to be easy to follow, using readily available ingredients. Each recipe includes detailed instructions, nutritional information, and helpful tips to make your cooking experience enjoyable and stress-free.

**Key Features:**

1. Nutrient-Packed Ingredients: Our recipes incorporate ingredients rich in heart-healthy nutrients like fiber, omega-3 fatty acids, and antioxidants.

2. Flavorful and Satisfying: You don't have to sacrifice taste for health. These recipes are full of flavor and will keep you satisfied throughout the morning.

3. Dietary Variety: We offer recipes suitable for different dietary preferences, including vegetarian and vegan options.

4. Nutritional Information: Each recipe provides essential nutritional information, helping you make informed choices.

5. Cooking Tips: We include valuable tips and techniques to make your cooking experience a success, even for beginners.

Get ready to embark on a delicious journey towards better heart health with our Breakfast Recipe Section. Start your day right and take a step closer to achieving optimal health and longevity. Remember, your heart will thank you for making these nutritious and tasty choices.

# Recipe 1: Sunrise Berry Smoothie Bowl

*Prep Time: 10 mins - No Cooking - Serves: 1*

**Ingredients:**

- 1 cup mixed frozen berries (strawberries, blueberries, raspberries)
- 1 frozen banana, sliced
- 1/2 cup Greek yogurt
- 1/2 cup almond milk or any milk of choice
- 1 tablespoon almond butter
- 1 tablespoon chia seeds
- Optional toppings: Sliced fresh fruit, granola, coconut flakes

**Instructions:**

1. In a blender, combine the mixed frozen berries, frozen banana, Greek yogurt, and almond milk. Blend until smooth and creamy.
2. Pour the smoothie mixture into a bowl.
3. Drizzle almond butter over the top of the smoothie.
4. Sprinkle chia seeds evenly across the bowl.
5. If desired, add additional toppings like sliced fresh fruit, granola, or coconut flakes for extra texture and flavor.
6. Serve immediately and enjoy a nutritious and energizing breakfast.

**Nutritional Facts:**

- Calories: 350
- Total Fat: 15g
- Total Carbs: 45g
- Fiber: 10g
- Net Carbs: 35g
- Protein: 15g

**Cooking Tip**: *For a thicker smoothie bowl, use less milk or add a handful of ice to the blender. You can also freeze the Greek yogurt in an ice cube tray beforehand for an even creamier texture. Experiment with different combinations of frozen fruits to vary the flavor profile.*

# Recipe 2: Savory Scrambled Tofu with Spinach and Tomatoes

*Prep Time: 10 mins - Cooking Time: 10 mins - Serves: 2*

**Ingredients:**
- 1 block (14 oz) firm tofu, drained and crumbled
- 2 tablespoons olive oil
- 1 small onion, chopped
- 2 garlic cloves, minced
- 1 cup fresh spinach, chopped
- 1 cup cherry tomatoes, halved
- 1/2 teaspoon turmeric powder
- Salt and pepper to taste
- Optional: Red pepper flakes, nutritional yeast, or fresh herbs for added flavor

**Instructions:**
1. Heat olive oil in a large skillet over medium heat. Add the chopped onion and minced garlic, sautéing until the onion is translucent.
2. Add the crumbled tofu to the skillet. Cook, stirring frequently, for about 5 minutes or until the tofu starts to turn golden.
3. Stir in the turmeric powder, salt, and pepper. Mix well to evenly coat the tofu.
4. Add the chopped spinach and cherry tomatoes to the skillet. Continue cooking for an additional 3-4 minutes or until the spinach wilts and the tomatoes soften.
5. If desired, sprinkle red pepper flakes, nutritional yeast, or fresh herbs over the scramble for extra flavor.
6. Serve the savory scrambled tofu hot, either on its own or with whole-grain toast for a complete meal.

**Nutritional Facts:**
- Calories: 250
- Total Fat: 18g
- Total Carbs: 10g
- Fiber: 3g
- Net Carbs: 7g
- Protein: 15g

**Cooking Tip:** *Pressing the tofu before cooking removes excess moisture and helps it absorb flavors better. This dish is highly customizable; you can add other vegetables like bell peppers or mushrooms. For a cheesy flavor without the dairy, sprinkle some nutritional yeast on top before serving.*

# Recipe 3: Overnight Oats with Cinnamon Apples and Walnuts

*Prep Time: 15 mins - No Cooking - Serves: 2*

**Ingredients:**

- 1 cup rolled oats
- 1 1/2 cups almond milk or any plant-based milk
- 1 tablespoon chia seeds
- 2 tablespoons maple syrup or honey
- 1 teaspoon ground cinnamon
- 1 apple, diced
- 1/4 cup walnuts, chopped

**Instructions:**

1. In a medium bowl or jar, combine the rolled oats, almond milk, chia seeds, maple syrup or honey, and ground cinnamon. Stir well until all ingredients are thoroughly mixed.

2. Cover the bowl or jar and refrigerate overnight, allowing the oats to soak and soften.

3. In the morning, give the oats a good stir. If the mixture is too thick, add a little more almond milk to reach your desired consistency.

4. Top the overnight oats with diced apples and chopped walnuts just before serving.

5. Serve the overnight oats cold or at room temperature for a nutritious and convenient breakfast.

**Nutritional Facts:**

- Calories: 350
- Total Fat: 12g
- Total Carbs: 52g
- Fiber: 8g
- Net Carbs: 44g
- Protein: 10g

**Cooking Tip:** *For added flavor and sweetness, you can sauté the diced apples in a little butter or coconut oil with extra cinnamon before adding them to the oats. You can also add a dollop of Greek yogurt or a spoonful of nut butter for extra protein. This recipe is versatile, and you can experiment with different fruits and nuts according to your preference.*

# Recipe 4: Mediterranean Avocado Toast with Poached Egg

*Prep Time: 15 mins - Cooking Time: 5 mins - Serves: 1*

## Ingredients:
- 1 ripe avocado
- 1 slice of whole-wheat bread
- 1 egg
- 1 tablespoon white vinegar (for poaching the egg)
- 2 tablespoons olive oil
- Salt and pepper to taste
- Fresh herbs (such as basil, parsley, or dill), finely chopped
- Optional: Red pepper flakes, lemon zest, or a sprinkle of feta cheese

## Instructions:
1. Bring a pot of water to a gentle simmer and add the white vinegar.
2. Crack the egg into a small bowl, then gently slide it into the simmering water. Poach for about 3-4 minutes for a soft yolk or longer for a firmer yolk. Remove the egg with a slotted spoon and set aside on a paper towel.
3. Toast the whole-wheat bread to your liking.
4. Mash the avocado in a bowl and season with salt and pepper.
5. Spread the mashed avocado evenly over the toasted bread.
6. Carefully place the poached egg on top of the avocado.
7. Drizzle with olive oil and sprinkle with fresh herbs. If desired, add red pepper flakes, lemon zest, or a sprinkle of feta cheese for extra flavor.
8. Serve immediately for a healthy and satisfying Mediterranean-inspired breakfast or snack.

## Nutritional Facts:
- Calories: 400
- Total Fat: 30g
- Total Carbs: 27g
- Fiber: 10g
- Net Carbs: 17g
- Protein: 14g

**Cooking Tip:** *For an even creamier texture, blend the avocado with a little Greek yogurt or cream cheese. If you're new to poaching eggs, using fresh eggs will help them hold their shape better in the water. This recipe is highly versatile, and you can customize it with additional toppings like smoked salmon, cherry tomatoes, or sliced cucumber.*

# Recipe 5: Greek Yogurt Parfait with Berries and Flaxseed Granola

*Prep Time: 15 mins - No Cooking - Serves: 1*

## Ingredients:

- 1 cup Greek yogurt
- 1/2 cup mixed berries (such as strawberries, blueberries, raspberries)
- 1/2 cup homemade or store-bought granola with flaxseeds
- Optional: Honey or maple syrup for sweetness, a sprinkle of chia seeds, or a dash of cinnamon

## Instructions:

1. In a serving glass or bowl, start by layering half of the Greek yogurt at the bottom.

2. Add a layer of mixed berries over the yogurt.

3. Sprinkle half of the granola with flaxseeds on top of the berries.

4. Repeat the layers with the remaining yogurt, berries, and granola.

5. If desired, drizzle a bit of honey or maple syrup over the top for added sweetness.

6. Optionally, sprinkle chia seeds or a dash of cinnamon on top for extra flavor and nutrition.

7. Serve the Greek yogurt parfait immediately as a healthy and filling breakfast or snack.

## Nutritional Facts:

- Calories: 350
- Total Fat: 10g
- Total Carbs: 45g
- Fiber: 6g
- Net Carbs: 39g
- Protein: 25g

**Cooking Tip:** *You can make your own granola with oats, flaxseeds, nuts, and a sweetener of your choice, baked until crispy. For a vegan version, use plant-based yogurt. This parfait can be customized with different types of fruit, nuts, or seeds according to your preference. If you prepare this ahead of time, keep the granola separate until just before serving to maintain its crunch.*

# Recipe 6: Baked Sweet Potato Hash with Black Beans and Salsa

*Prep Time: 15 mins - Cooking Time: 30 mins - Serves: 2*

## Ingredients:

- 2 large sweet potatoes, peeled and diced
- 1 tablespoon olive oil
- 1 can (15 ounces) black beans, drained and rinsed
- Salt and pepper to taste
- 1/2 teaspoon smoked paprika (optional)
- 1/2 cup fresh salsa
- Optional: Chopped cilantro, avocado slices, or a dollop of Greek yogurt for garnish

## Instructions:

1. Preheat the oven to 400°F (200°C).

2. In a large bowl, toss the diced sweet potatoes with olive oil, salt, pepper, and smoked paprika if using. Spread the sweet potatoes in a single layer on a baking sheet.

3. Roast in the oven for 20 minutes, stirring halfway through, until the sweet potatoes are tender and starting to brown.

4. Add the black beans to the baking sheet with the sweet potatoes. Stir to combine and roast for an additional 10 minutes.

5. To serve, divide the sweet potato and black bean mixture between plates. Top each serving with a generous spoonful of fresh salsa.

6. Garnish with chopped cilantro, avocado slices, or a dollop of Greek yogurt if desired.

## Nutritional Facts:

- Calories: 330
- Total Fat: 7g
- Total Carbs: 58g
- Fiber: 13g
- Net Carbs: 45g
- Protein: 10g

**Cooking Tip:** *For a heartier meal, you can add diced bell peppers or onions to the sweet potatoes before roasting. The salsa can be homemade or store-bought; choose a fresh, chunky variety for the best flavor and texture. This dish can be served as a filling breakfast, a satisfying lunch, or even a casual dinner. The combination of sweet potatoes and black beans provides a good balance of complex carbohydrates, fiber, and protein.*

# Recipe 7: Chia Seed Pudding with Mango and Coconut Milk

*Prep Time: 15 mins - No Cooking - Serves: 2*

## Ingredients:

- 1/4 cup chia seeds
- 1 cup coconut milk
- 1 tablespoon honey or maple syrup (optional)
- 1 teaspoon vanilla extract
- 1 ripe mango, diced
- Optional: Shredded coconut or sliced almonds for garnish

## Instructions:

1. In a medium bowl, whisk together the chia seeds, coconut milk, honey or maple syrup (if using), and vanilla extract until well combined.

2. Divide the mixture between two serving glasses or bowls. Cover and refrigerate for at least 2 hours, or overnight, until the pudding has thickened and the chia seeds have absorbed the coconut milk.

3. Once the chia pudding has set, layer the diced mango on top of each serving.

4. If desired, garnish with shredded coconut or sliced almonds for added texture and flavor.

5. Serve the chia seed pudding chilled as a refreshing and nutritious breakfast or snack.

## Nutritional Facts:

- Calories: 300
- Total Fat: 18g
- Total Carbs: 30g
- Fiber: 9g
- Net Carbs: 21g
- Protein: 5g

**Cooking Tip:** *For a smoother texture, you can blend the chia pudding after it has set. Adjust the sweetness to your liking by adding more or less honey or maple syrup. You can also layer the pudding with additional fruits like pineapple or berries for extra flavor and color. This pudding is not only healthy but also versatile, making it a perfect option for meal prep or a quick on-the-go snack.*

# Recipe 8: Whole-Wheat Pancakes with Banana and Blueberries

*Prep Time: 15 mins - Cooking Time: 10 mins - Serves: 4*

## Ingredients:

- 1 1/2 cups whole-wheat flour
- 2 tablespoons sugar (optional)
- 1 tablespoon baking powder
- 1/2 teaspoon salt
- 1 1/4 cups milk
- 1 large egg
- 1 tablespoon vegetable oil or melted butter
- 1 teaspoon vanilla extract
- 2 bananas, sliced
- 1 cup blueberries (fresh or frozen)
- Optional: Maple syrup or honey for serving

## Instructions:

1. In a large bowl, whisk together the whole-wheat flour, sugar (if using), baking powder, and salt.

2. In another bowl, beat the milk, egg, vegetable oil, melted butter, and vanilla extract together.

3. Pour the wet ingredients into the dry ingredients and stir until just combined. The batter should be slightly lumpy.

4. Heat a non-stick skillet or griddle over medium heat. Lightly grease with oil or butter.

5. Pour about 1/4 cup of batter for each pancake onto the skillet. Cook until bubbles appear on the surface, then flip and cook until golden brown on the other side.

6. Top the pancakes with sliced bananas and blueberries.

7. Serve warm, with maple syrup or honey if desired.

## Nutritional Facts:

- Calories: 280
- Total Fat: 6g
- Total Carbs: 50g
- Fiber: 7g
- Net Carbs: 43g
- Protein: 9g

**Cooking Tip:** *For extra fluffy pancakes, let the batter rest for 5-10 minutes before cooking. You can also add the blueberries directly to the batter if preferred. For a dairy-free version, use almond milk or another plant-based milk. These whole-wheat pancakes are a great way to start your day with a nutritious and satisfying meal.*

# Recipe 9: Turkey Sausage and Veggie Scramble

*Prep Time - 15 minutes - Cooking Time - 10 minutes - Servings – 4*

**Ingredients:**

- 8 oz lean turkey sausage, casing removed and crumbled
- 1 small onion, diced
- 1 red bell pepper, diced
- 1 green bell pepper, diced
- 1 cup spinach, chopped
- 8 large eggs
- 1/4 cup milk
- 1/2 teaspoon salt
- 1/4 teaspoon black pepper
- 1/4 cup cheddar cheese, shredded (optional)
- 1 tablespoon olive oil

**Cooking Instructions:**

1. Heat the olive oil in a large skillet over medium heat. Add the crumbled turkey sausage and cook until browned, about 5 minutes.
2. Add the diced onion and bell peppers to the skillet with the sausage. Cook until the vegetables are soft, about 3-4 minutes.
3. Stir in the chopped spinach and cook until wilted, about 2 minutes.
4. In a bowl, whisk together the eggs, milk, salt, and pepper. Pour this mixture over the sausage and vegetables in the skillet.
5. Allow the eggs to set around the edges, then gently stir to combine with the sausage and vegetables. Cook until the eggs are fully set but still moist.
6. If using, sprinkle shredded cheddar cheese over the scramble. Let it melt for about 1 minute.
7. Serve the turkey sausage and veggie scramble hot.

**Top 5 Nutritional Values:**

- Calories: 280 kcal per serving
- Fiber: 2 g per serving
- Healthy Fats: 18 g per serving (with cheese)
- Protein: 23 g per serving
- Vitamin C: Excellent source due to bell peppers

**Cooking Tip:** *For a lighter version, you can use egg whites instead of whole eggs. Feel free to add other vegetables like mushrooms or zucchini to the scramble for added flavor and nutrition. This dish is a versatile breakfast that can be easily adapted to your taste preferences.*

# Recipe 10: Eggless Pumpkin Muffins with Maple Pecan Topping

*Prep Time: 20 minutes  - Cooking Time:\*\* 25 minutes  - Serves: 12 muffins*

## Ingredients:

- 1 1/2 cups gluten-free all-purpose flour
- 1 tsp baking soda
- 1/2 tsp salt
- 1 tsp ground cinnamon
- 1/2 tsp ground ginger
- 1/4 tsp ground nutmeg
- 1/4 tsp ground cloves
- 1 cup pumpkin puree
- 3/4 cup brown sugar
- 1/2 cup vegetable oil
- 1/4 cup maple syrup
- 1/4 cup almond milk
- 1 tsp vanilla extract

## For the Maple Pecan Topping:

- 1/2 cup chopped pecans
- 2 tbsp gluten-free all-purpose flour
- 2 tbsp brown sugar
- 1 tbsp melted butter
- 2 tbsp maple syrup

## Cooking Instructions:

1. Preheat the oven to 350°F (175°C). Line a muffin tin with paper liners or lightly grease it.

2. In a bowl, whisk together the gluten-free flour, baking soda, salt, cinnamon, ginger, nutmeg, and cloves.

3. In another bowl, mix the pumpkin puree, brown sugar, vegetable oil, maple syrup, almond milk, and vanilla extract.

4. Combine the wet and dry ingredients, stirring until just mixed.

5. Fill each muffin cup about 3/4 full with the batter.

6. For the topping, mix the chopped pecans, gluten-free flour, brown sugar, melted butter, and maple syrup in a small bowl. Sprinkle this mixture over the muffin batter.

7. Bake for 25 minutes or until a toothpick inserted into the center comes out clean.

8. Allow to cool before serving.

## Nutritional Facts:

- Calories: 210
- Total Fat: 11g
- Total Carbs: 28g
- Fiber: 2g
- Net Carbs: 26g
- Protein: 3g

**Cooking Tip:** *For extra moisture and flavor, try adding a tablespoon of orange zest to the muffin batter. It pairs wonderfully with the pumpkin and spices!*

# Chapter 11: Delicious and Heart-Healthy Lunch Recipes for Lower Cholesterol and Triglycerides

Embrace a midday meal that nourishes your heart and tantalizes your taste buds with "10 Delicious and Heart-Healthy Lunch Recipes for Lower Cholesterol and Triglycerides." This chapter is designed for those who seek to balance delectable flavors with the benefits of a heart-healthy diet. Lunchtime is a crucial part of your day, and these recipes ensure that it's not just a meal but a delightful and healthy experience.

Focused on ingredients known to support heart health and lower cholesterol and triglyceride levels, each recipe in this chapter is a step towards a healthier, happier heart. These meals are crafted to be low in saturated fats and rich in nutrients like fiber, healthy fats, and antioxidants, making them perfect for anyone looking to improve their cardiovascular health through diet.

Dive into a selection of lunch recipes that are both satisfying and conducive to maintaining a healthy heart. These dishes are thoughtfully created to be easy to prepare, delicious, and beneficial in managing cholesterol and triglycerides.

Each recipe in this chapter is a blend of delicious flavors and heart-healthy ingredients, proving that food that's good for your heart can also delight your palate. These lunch recipes are perfect for anyone looking to enjoy a midday meal that supports their cardiovascular health and keeps their taste buds happy.

# Recipe 11: Mediterranean Quinoa Salad with Chickpeas and Grilled Vegetables

*Prep Time: 15 minutes - Cooking Time: 20 minutes - Serves: 4*

## Ingredients:

- 1 cup quinoa, rinsed
- 2 cups water
- 1 can (15 oz) chickpeas, drained and rinsed
- 1 medium zucchini, sliced
- 1 red bell pepper, cut into strips
- 1 yellow bell pepper, cut into strips
- 1/4 cup olive oil, divided
- Salt and pepper, to taste
- 1/4 cup tahini
- Juice of 1 lemon
- 2 cloves garlic, minced
- 2 tbsp fresh parsley, chopped
- 1 tsp paprika
- 1/4 cup crumbled feta cheese (optional)

## Cooking Instructions:

1. In a saucepan, combine quinoa and water. Bring to a boil, then reduce heat to low, cover, and simmer for 15 minutes until quinoa is cooked and water is absorbed.

2. While the quinoa is cooking, preheat the grill or a grill pan over medium heat.

3. Toss zucchini and bell peppers with 2 tablespoons of olive oil, salt, and pepper. Grill the vegetables until tender and slightly charred, about 3-4 minutes per side.

4. In a small bowl, whisk together tahini, lemon juice, remaining olive oil, garlic, parsley, and paprika to make the dressing.

5. In a large bowl, combine cooked quinoa, grilled vegetables, chickpeas, and dressing. Toss well to combine.

6. Sprinkle with feta cheese if using, and serve.

## Nutritional Facts:

- Calories: 320
- Total Fat: 14g
- Total Carbs: 42g
- Fiber: 8g
- Net Carbs: 34g
- Protein: 12g

**Cooking Tip:** *For added crunch and nutrition, include a handful of chopped raw red onion and cucumber in the salad. They add a fresh, crisp texture and complement the flavors of the grilled vegetables.*

# Recipe 12: Spicy Salmon Lettuce Wraps with Avocado and Cilantro

*Prep Time: 20 minutes  -  Cooking Time: 10 minutes  -  Serves: 4*

**Ingredients:**
- 4 salmon fillets (about 6 ounces each)
- 1 tbsp olive oil
- 1 tsp chili powder
- 1/2 tsp cumin
- Salt and pepper, to taste
- 1 large head of butter lettuce, leaves separated
- 2 ripe avocados, sliced
- 1/4 cup fresh cilantro leaves

**For the Zesty Salsa:**
- 2 medium tomatoes, finely chopped
- 1 small red onion, finely chopped
- 1 jalapeño, seeded and minced
- Juice of 1 lime
- Salt and pepper, to taste

**Cooking Instructions:**
1. Preheat your grill or a grill pan over medium-high heat.
2. Rub each salmon fillet with olive oil and season with chili powder, cumin, salt, and pepper.
3. Grill the salmon for about 5 minutes on each side or until cooked through and flaky.
4. While the salmon is cooking, prepare the zesty salsa by combining tomatoes, red onion, jalapeño, lime juice, salt, and pepper in a bowl. Set aside.
5. To assemble the wraps, place a salmon fillet on each lettuce leaf, add slices of avocado, and sprinkle with cilantro leaves.
6. Top each wrap with a spoonful of the zesty salsa.
7. Serve immediately, as the lettuce leaves will remain crisp.

**Nutritional Facts:**
- Calories: 290
- Total Fat: 17g
- Total Carbs: 9g
- Fiber: 4g
- Net Carbs: 5g
- Protein: 27g

**Cooking Tip:** *For an extra kick, marinate the salmon fillets in a mixture of olive oil, lime juice, and a bit of sriracha or your favorite hot sauce for 30 minutes before grilling. This will infuse the salmon with spicy flavors that complement the coolness of the lettuce and avocado.*

# Recipe 13: Lentil and Vegetable Soup with Whole-Wheat Croutons

*Prep Time: 15 minutes  -  Cooking Time: 45 minutes  -  Serves: 6*

**Ingredients:**
- 1 cup dried lentils, rinsed
- 2 tablespoons olive oil
- 1 onion, chopped
- 2 carrots, diced
- 2 celery stalks, diced
- 3 garlic cloves, minced
- 1 zucchini, diced
- 1 red bell pepper, diced
- 1 teaspoon ground turmeric
- 6 cups vegetable broth
- Salt and pepper, to taste
- 1 can (14.5 oz) diced tomatoes
- 2 cups spinach leaves

**For the Whole-Wheat Croutons:**
- 4 slices whole-wheat bread, cubed
- 2 tablespoons olive oil
- 1/2 teaspoon garlic powder
- 1/2 teaspoon dried parsley

**Cooking Instructions:**
1. In a large pot, heat olive oil over medium heat. Add onion, carrots, celery, and garlic. Cook until vegetables are tender, about 5 minutes.
2. Add zucchini, red bell pepper, and turmeric, cooking for another 2 minutes.
3. Add lentils and vegetable broth. Bring to a boil, then reduce heat and simmer for 30 minutes or until lentils are tender.
4. While the soup is simmering, make the croutons. Preheat oven to 375°F (190°C). Toss bread cubes with olive oil, garlic powder, and dried parsley. Spread on a baking sheet and bake for 10-15 minutes, until crisp and golden.
5. Add diced tomatoes and spinach to the soup, cooking until spinach is wilted. Season with salt and pepper.
6. Serve the soup hot, topped with whole-wheat croutons.

**Nutritional Facts:**
- Calories: 220
- Total Fat: 5g
- Total Carbs: 33g
- Fiber: 11g
- Net Carbs: 22g
- Protein: 12g

**Cooking Tip:** *For a creamier texture, blend a portion of the soup before adding the spinach and tomatoes. This adds a rich, smooth consistency to the soup while maintaining the hearty feel of the lentils and vegetables.*

# Recipe 14: Black Bean and Mango Tostadas

*Prep Time: 20 minutes  -  Cooking Time: 5 minutes  -  Serves: 4*

## Ingredients:

- 4 whole wheat or corn tortillas
- 1 can (15 oz) black beans, drained and rinsed
- 1 ripe mango, peeled and diced
- 1 small red onion, finely chopped
- Juice of 1 lime
- Salt and pepper, to taste
- 1/4 cup fresh cilantro, chopped
- 1 avocado, sliced (optional)
- 1/4 cup crumbled feta cheese (optional)

## Cooking Instructions:

1. Preheat the oven to 400°F (200°C). Place tortillas on a baking sheet and bake for 3-5 minutes or until crisp.

2. Mash the black beans in a bowl with a fork. Spread the mashed beans evenly over each crisp tortilla.

3. Top with diced mango, red onion, and a sprinkle of lime juice. Add salt and pepper to taste.

4. Garnish with chopped cilantro, avocado slices, and feta cheese if using.

5. Serve immediately while the tortillas are still crispy.

## Nutritional Facts:

- Calories: 260
- Total Fat: 6g
- Total Carbs: 42g
- Fiber: 10g
- Net Carbs: 32g
- Protein: 10g

**Cooking Tip:** *To add a spicy kick, drizzle a bit of hot sauce or sprinkle some chili flakes on top of the tostadas. This contrasts nicely with the sweetness of the mango and the creaminess of the avocado.*

# Recipe 15: Tuna Salad with Greek Yogurt and Lemon Dill

*Prep Time: 10 mins - No Cooking - Serves: 4*

**Ingredients:**

- 2 cans (5 oz each) of tuna in water, drained
- 1/2 cup Greek yogurt
- 1 tablespoon fresh dill, chopped
- Zest and juice of 1 lemon
- 1/4 cup red onion, finely chopped
- 1/4 cup celery, finely chopped
- Salt and pepper, to taste
- Whole-wheat bread or crackers for serving

**Instructions:**

1. In a mixing bowl, flake the tuna with a fork.

2. Add Greek yogurt, dill, lemon zest, lemon juice, red onion, and celery to the bowl. Mix thoroughly until combined.

3. Season the tuna salad with salt and pepper according to your taste preference.

4. The tuna salad can be served on whole-wheat bread for a satisfying sandwich or with crackers for a light snack.

**Nutritional Facts:**

- Calories: 140
- Total Fat: 2g
- Total Carbs: 4g
- Fiber: 1g
- Net Carbs: 3g
- Protein: 24g

**Cooking Tip:** *To add a refreshing and crunchy texture to your tuna salad, consider including chopped cucumbers or radishes. This not only provides an enjoyable crunch but also enhances the nutritional value of your meal.*

# Recipe 16: Veggie Powerhouse Pita Pockets

*Prep Time: 20 mins - Cooking Time: 25 mins - Serves: 4*

## Ingredients:

- 2 large sweet potatoes, peeled and diced
- 4 portobello mushroom caps
- 4 whole-wheat pita pockets
- 1 cup hummus
- 2 cups fresh spinach
- 1/4 cup tahini
- 2 tablespoons olive oil
- Salt and pepper, to taste
- Optional: sliced avocado or cucumber

## Instructions:

1. Preheat the oven to 400°F (200°C).

2. Toss the diced sweet potatoes with 1 tablespoon olive oil, salt, and pepper. Spread them on a baking sheet and roast for 20 minutes or until tender.

3. While the sweet potatoes are roasting, brush the portobello mushrooms with the remaining olive oil and season with salt and pepper. Grill them on a grill pan over medium heat on each side for about 5 minutes.

4. To assemble, cut each pita pocket in half and spread hummus inside each half.

5. Stuff the pita pockets with roasted sweet potatoes, grilled portobello mushrooms, and fresh spinach. Drizzle tahini over the filling.

6. If desired, add sliced avocado or cucumber for extra freshness and crunch.

7. Serve immediately while the vegetables are still warm.

## Nutritional Facts:

- Calories: 390
- Total Fat: 17g
- Total Carbs: 52g
- Fiber: 10g
- Net Carbs: 42g
- Protein: 12g

**Cooking Tip:** *For a smoky flavor, sprinkle some smoked paprika on the sweet potatoes before roasting. This adds a delightful depth to the overall taste of the pita pockets.*

# Recipe 17: Quinoa Tabouli Salad with Grilled Chicken

*Prep Time: 20 mins - Cooking Time: 15 mins - Serves: 4*

**Ingredients:**

- 1 cup quinoa, rinsed
- 2 cups water
- 2 boneless, skinless chicken breasts
- 2 cups fresh parsley, finely chopped
- 1/2 cup fresh mint, finely chopped
- 2 large tomatoes, diced
- 1 cucumber, diced
- Juice of 2 lemons
- 1/4 cup olive oil
- Salt and pepper, to taste
- Optional: crumbled feta cheese

**Instructions:**

1. In a saucepan, bring the quinoa and water to a boil. Reduce the heat, cover, and simmer for 15 minutes or until the water is absorbed. Fluff the quinoa with a fork and let it cool.

2. Season the chicken breasts with salt and pepper. Grill them over medium heat for about 7 minutes per side or until cooked through. Let them rest for a few minutes, then slice them.

3. In a large bowl, combine the cooled quinoa, parsley, mint, tomatoes, and cucumber.

4. In a small bowl, whisk together lemon juice and olive oil. Pour this dressing over the salad and toss well.

5. Season the tabouli salad with salt and pepper.

6. Serve the salad with sliced grilled chicken on top. Add crumbled feta cheese if desired.

**Nutritional Facts:**

- Calories: 320
- Total Fat: 10g
- Total Carbs: 35g
- Fiber: 6g
- Net Carbs: 29g
- Protein: 22g

**Cooking Tip:** *To infuse the quinoa with more flavor, cook it in chicken or vegetable broth instead of water. This adds an extra layer of savory taste to the tabouli salad.*

# Recipe 18: Turkey and Avocado Roll-Ups with Sprouts

*Prep Time: 10 mins - No Cooking - Serves: 4*

## Ingredients:

- 8 slices of turkey breast (thinly sliced)
- 2 ripe avocados, sliced
- 1 cup alfalfa sprouts
- 4 tablespoons Dijon mustard
- Salt and pepper, to taste
- Optional: whole wheat tortillas or lettuce leaves for wrapping

## Instructions:

1. Lay out the turkey slices on a flat surface.

2. Spread a thin layer of Dijon mustard on each turkey slice.

3. Place a few slices of avocado and a small handful of alfalfa sprouts on each slice.

4. Season with salt and pepper.

5. Carefully roll up each turkey slice, enclosing the avocado and sprouts.

6. If using, wrap each roll-up in a whole wheat tortilla or a lettuce leaf for easier handling and added nutrients.

7. Serve immediately or chill in the refrigerator until ready to eat.

## Nutritional Facts:

- Calories: 180
- Total Fat: 9g
- Total Carbs: 6g
- Fiber: 4g
- Net Carbs: 2g
- Protein: 20g

**Cooking Tip:** *For a variation, add a thin slice of cheese or a spread of cream cheese inside the roll-ups for extra creaminess and flavor. You can also include thin slices of cucumber or bell pepper for added crunch.*

# Recipe 19: Mediterranean Chickpea Salad Sandwich

*Prep Time: 15 mins - No Cooking - Serves: 4*

**Ingredients:**

- 1 can (15 oz) chickpeas, drained and rinsed
- 1/4 cup sun-dried tomatoes, chopped
- 1/4 cup olives, pitted and chopped
- 2 tablespoons fresh parsley, chopped
- 1 tablespoon fresh basil, chopped
- Juice of 1 lemon
- 2 tablespoons olive oil
- Salt and pepper, to taste
- 8 slices whole-wheat bread
- 4 lettuce leaves
- 1 large tomato, sliced

**Instructions:**

1. In a bowl, mash the chickpeas with a fork until slightly chunky.

2. Add the sun-dried tomatoes, olives, parsley, basil, lemon juice, and olive oil to the mashed chickpeas. Mix until well combined. Season with salt and pepper.

3. Spread the chickpea salad evenly over 4 slices of whole-wheat bread.

4. Add a lettuce leaf and a couple of tomato slices to each sandwich.

5. Top with the remaining slices of bread.

6. Cut each sandwich in half and serve.

**Nutritional Facts:**

- Calories: 350
- Total Fat: 12g
- Total Carbs: 50g
- Fiber: 12g
- Net Carbs: 38g
- Protein: 14g

**Cooking Tip:** *For a creamier texture, you can add a dollop of Greek yogurt or hummus to the chickpea mixture. This adds moisture and a tangy flavor to the sandwich.*

# Recipe 20: Thai Coconut Curry Noodle Soup with Tofu

*Prep Time: 20 mins - Cooking Time: 30 mins - Serves: 4*

**Ingredients:**

- 200g rice noodles
- 1 tablespoon coconut oil
- 1 onion, thinly sliced
- 2 cloves garlic, minced
- 1 tablespoon fresh ginger, grated
- 1 red bell pepper, thinly sliced
- 1 carrot, julienned
- 1 tablespoon red curry paste
- 400ml can of coconut milk
- 4 cups vegetable broth
- 1 tablespoon soy sauce
- 1 tablespoon lime juice
- 200g firm tofu, cubed
- 1 cup baby spinach
- Fresh cilantro and sliced red chili for garnish

**Instructions:**

1. Prepare the rice noodles according to the package instructions, then drain and set aside.
2. In a large pot, heat the coconut oil over medium heat. Add the onion, garlic, and ginger, sautéing until the onion is translucent.
3. Add the red bell pepper and carrot, cooking for a few minutes until they start to soften.
4. Stir in the red curry paste, then pour in the coconut milk and vegetable broth. Bring to a simmer.
5. Add the soy sauce and lime juice to the soup, adjusting the seasoning to taste.
6. Add the tofu and simmer for about 10 minutes to absorb the flavors.
7. Stir in the baby spinach until it wilts.
8. To serve, divide the rice noodles among bowls, pour the hot soup over them, and garnish with cilantro and red chili slices.

**Nutritional Facts:**

- Calories: 350
- Total Fat: 14g
- Total Carbs: 45g
- Fiber: 3g
- Net Carbs: 42g
- Protein: 12g

**Cooking Tip:** *For added depth and complexity in the broth, you can include a stalk of lemongrass (bruised and cut into large pieces) and a few kaffir lime leaves. Remove these before serving for a more authentic Thai flavor experience.*

# Chapter 12: Delicious and Heart-Healthy Dinner Recipes for Lower Cholesterol and Triglycerides

Embark on a culinary journey that promises both delectable flavors and a healthier heart with "10 Delicious and Heart-Healthy Dinner Recipes for Lower Cholesterol and Triglycerides." This chapter is a treasure trove for anyone aiming to manage their cholesterol and triglyceride levels without compromising on taste. It's a fusion of culinary creativity and nutritional wisdom designed to bring heart-healthy eating right to your dinner table.

Eating for heart health doesn't have to be bland or restrictive. The recipes in this chapter are carefully crafted to be rich in nutrients that are beneficial for maintaining healthy cholesterol and triglyceride levels. They focus on incorporating a variety of ingredients known for their heart-healthy properties, such as lean proteins, whole grains, and an abundance of fruits and vegetables.

In this chapter, we present ten dinner recipes that are not just mouth-watering but also align with a heart-healthy dietary pattern. These meals are tailored to be low in unhealthy fats and high in fiber and other beneficial nutrients, helping you to manage your cholesterol and triglycerides effectively.

Each recipe in this chapter is designed to bring you the best of both worlds: a festival of flavors and a boost to your heart health. These meals are ideal for anyone looking to enjoy delicious dinners while keeping an eye on their cholesterol and triglyceride levels. Enjoy these recipes as part of your journey towards a healthier heart.

# Recipe 21: Baked Salmon with Lemon Dill Sauce and Roasted Asparagus

*Prep Time: 15 mins - Cooking Time: 20 mins - Serves: 4*

## Ingredients:

- 4 salmon fillets (about 6 ounces each)
- 1 bunch asparagus, ends trimmed
- 2 tablespoons olive oil, divided
- Salt and pepper, to taste
- 1 lemon, juiced and zested
- 2 tablespoons fresh dill, chopped
- 1 garlic clove, minced
- 1/4 cup Greek yogurt
- 1 tablespoon Dijon mustard

## Instructions:

1. Preheat the oven to 400°F (200°C). Line a baking sheet with parchment paper.

2. Place the salmon fillets on one side of the prepared baking sheet.

3. On the other side, lay out the asparagus and drizzle with 1 tablespoon of olive oil. Season with salt and pepper.

4. In a small bowl, mix together lemon juice and zest, dill, garlic, Greek yogurt, and Dijon mustard. Season with salt and pepper to taste.

5. Spread the lemon dill sauce evenly over each salmon fillet.

6. Drizzle the remaining olive oil over the salmon.

7. Bake in the preheated oven for about 15-20 minutes, or until the salmon is cooked through and the asparagus is tender.

8. Serve the baked salmon with the roasted asparagus on the side.

## Nutritional Facts:

- Calories: 300
- Total Fat: 15g
- Total Carbs: 6g
- Fiber: 2g
- Net Carbs: 4g
- Protein: 35g

**Cooking Tip:** *For an extra crispy texture on the asparagus, broil them for the last 2-3 minutes of cooking. This will give them a nice char and enhance their flavor.*

# Recipe 22: Mediterranean Chicken Kebabs with Greek Yogurt Marinade

*Prep Time: 30 mins (plus marinating time) - Cooking Time: 15 mins - Serves: 4*

## Ingredients:

- 4 boneless, skinless chicken breasts cut into cubes
- 1 cup Greek yogurt
- 2 cloves garlic, minced
- 2 tablespoons olive oil
- Juice of 1 lemon
- 1 tablespoon dried oregano
- 1 teaspoon paprika
- Salt and pepper, to taste
- 1 red bell pepper, cut into chunks
- 1 zucchini, sliced into rounds
- 1 onion, cut into chunks
- 1 cup couscous, cooked according to package instructions

## Instructions:

1. In a large bowl, combine Greek yogurt, garlic, olive oil, lemon juice, oregano, paprika, salt, and pepper.

2. Add the chicken cubes to the marinade, ensuring they are well coated. Cover and refrigerate for at least 2 hours, preferably overnight.

3. Preheat the grill to medium-high heat.

4. Thread the marinated chicken, bell pepper, zucchini, and onion onto skewers.

5. Grill the kebabs, turning occasionally, until the chicken is cooked through and the vegetables are tender, about 10-15 minutes.

6. Serve the chicken kebabs with cooked couscous on the side.

## Nutritional Facts:

- Calories: 350
- Total Fat: 10g
- Total Carbs: 33g
- Fiber: 3g
- Net Carbs: 30g
- Protein: 30g

**Cooking Tip**: *To prevent wooden skewers from burning on the grill, soak them in water for at least 30 minutes before threading the chicken and vegetables. This will ensure even cooking without the skewers charring.*

# Recipe 23: Lentil Shepherd's Pie with Sweet Potato Mash

*Prep Time: 25 mins - Cooking Time: 30 mins - Serves: 6*

## Ingredients:

- 2 large sweet potatoes, peeled and cubed
- 1 tablespoon olive oil
- 1 onion, finely chopped
- 2 carrots, diced
- 2 celery stalks, diced
- 2 cloves garlic, minced
- 1 1/2 cups brown lentils, rinsed and drained
- 4 cups vegetable broth
- 1 teaspoon thyme
- 1 teaspoon rosemary
- Salt and pepper, to taste
- 1/2 cup milk (dairy or plant-based)
- 2 tablespoons butter (or vegan alternative)
- Optional: 1 cup frozen peas

## Instructions:

1. Preheat the oven to 375°F (190°C).
2. Boil sweet potatoes in a pot of water until tender, about 15 minutes. Drain and mash with milk and butter. Season with salt and pepper. Set aside.
3. In a large skillet, heat olive oil over medium heat. Add onion, carrots, and celery, and cook until softened, about 5 minutes. Add garlic and cook for another minute.
4. Stir in lentils, vegetable broth, thyme, and rosemary. Bring to a simmer and cook until the lentils are tender about 20 minutes. If using, add frozen peas in the last 5 minutes of cooking.
5. Season the lentil mixture with salt and pepper.
6. Transfer the lentil mixture to a baking dish. Top with the sweet potato mash, spreading it evenly.
7. Bake in the preheated oven for 25-30 minutes or until the top is slightly golden.
8. Let it cool for a few minutes before serving.

## Nutritional Facts:

- Calories: 320
- Total Fat: 6g
- Total Carbs: 54g
- Fiber: 14g
- Net Carbs: 40g
- Protein: 14g

**Cooking Tip***: For added richness and depth of flavor, consider adding a splash of red wine to the lentil mixture while cooking. This complements the earthiness of the lentils and the sweetness of the sweet potatoes.*

# Recipe 24: Shrimp Scampi with Zucchini Noodles

*Prep Time: 20 mins - Cooking Time: 10 mins - Serves: 4*

## Ingredients:

- 1 pound large shrimp, peeled and deveined
- 4 medium zucchini, spiralized into noodles
- 3 tablespoons olive oil
- 4 cloves garlic, minced
- 1/2 cup white wine
- Juice of 1 lemon
- 1/4 teaspoon red pepper flakes (optional)
- Salt and pepper, to taste
- 2 tablespoons fresh parsley, chopped
- Grated Parmesan cheese, for garnish (optional)

## Instructions:

1. Pat the shrimp dry with paper towels and season with salt and pepper.
2. Heat 2 tablespoons of olive oil in a large skillet over medium-high heat. Add the shrimp and cook for about 2 minutes on each side or until pink and opaque. Remove shrimp from the skillet and set aside.
3. In the same skillet, add the remaining tablespoon of olive oil and the garlic. Sauté for 1 minute until fragrant.
4. Add the white wine and lemon juice to the skillet, scraping up any browned bits from the bottom. Add red pepper flakes if using. Simmer for 2-3 minutes to reduce slightly.
5. Add the zucchini noodles to the skillet and toss to coat in the garlic-wine sauce. Cook for 2-3 minutes until the noodles are tender but still have a bit of crunch.
6. Return the shrimp to the skillet and toss to combine. Heat through for 1 minute.
7. Serve the shrimp and zucchini noodles garnished with chopped parsley and grated Parmesan cheese, if desired.

## Nutritional Facts:

- Calories: 250
- Total Fat: 10g
- Total Carbs: 10g
- Fiber: 2g
- Net Carbs: 8g
- Protein: 24g

**Cooking Tip**: *For an extra touch of flavor, finish the dish with a splash of good quality extra-virgin olive oil and a squeeze of fresh lemon juice right before serving. This enhances the freshness and brings all the flavors together beautifully.*

# Recipe 25: One-Pan Roasted Chicken and Vegetables with Lemon Herb Dressing

*Prep Time: 15 mins - Cooking Time: 35 mins - Serves: 4*

**Ingredients:**
- 4 boneless, skinless chicken breasts
- 2 carrots, peeled and sliced
- 1 red bell pepper, cut into chunks
- 1 zucchini, cut into chunks
- 1 yellow squash, cut into chunks
- 2 tablespoons olive oil
- Salt and pepper, to taste
- 1 teaspoon dried thyme
- 1 teaspoon dried rosemary

**For the Lemon Herb Dressing:**
- Juice of 1 lemon
- 1/4 cup olive oil
- 1 garlic clove, minced
- 1 tablespoon fresh parsley, chopped
- 1 teaspoon honey
- Salt and pepper, to taste

**Instructions:**
1. Preheat the oven to 425°F (220°C).
2. Arrange the chicken and vegetables in a single layer on a large baking sheet. Drizzle with 2 tablespoons of olive oil and season with salt, pepper, thyme, and rosemary. Toss to coat evenly.
3. Roast in the preheated oven for about 25-30 minutes, or until the chicken is cooked through and the vegetables are tender and slightly caramelized.
4. While the chicken and vegetables are roasting, prepare the lemon herb dressing. In a small bowl, whisk together lemon juice, olive oil, garlic, parsley, honey, salt, and pepper.
5. Once the chicken and vegetables are done, drizzle the lemon herb dressing over the top while everything is still warm.
6. Serve immediately, ensuring each plate gets a generous helping of both chicken and vegetables along with the dressing.

**Nutritional Facts:**
- Calories: 350
- Total Fat: 15g
- Total Carbs: 15g
- Fiber: 3g
- Net Carbs: 12g
- Protein: 35g

**Cooking Tip:** *For a deeper flavor, marinate the chicken in a mixture of olive oil, lemon juice, and herbs for at least an hour before roasting. This not only tenderizes the chicken but also infuses it with aromatic flavors that complement the roasted vegetables.*

# Recipe 26: Black Bean Burgers with Avocado and Chipotle Mayo

*Prep Time: 20 mins - Cooking Time: 10 mins - Serves: 4*

**Ingredients:**

- 2 cans (15 oz each) black beans, drained and rinsed
- 1/2 cup breadcrumbs
- 1/4 cup red onion, finely chopped
- 1 clove garlic, minced
- 1 teaspoon cumin
- 1/2 teaspoon smoked paprika
- Salt and pepper, to taste
- 1 egg (or flax egg for a vegan option)
- 2 tablespoons olive oil
- 4 whole-wheat burger buns
- 1 ripe avocado, sliced

**For the Chipotle Mayo:**

- 1/2 cup mayonnaise (or vegan alternative)
- 1 chipotle pepper in adobo sauce, finely chopped
- 1 tablespoon adobo sauce from the can
- Juice of 1/2 lime

**Instructions:**

1. In a large bowl, mash the black beans until mostly smooth.
2. Mix in breadcrumbs, red onion, garlic, cumin, smoked paprika, salt, and pepper. Stir in the egg until well combined.
3. Form the mixture into 4 burger patties.
4. Heat olive oil in a pan over medium heat. Cook the patties for about 5 minutes on each side or until they are heated through and have a crisp outer layer.
5. To make the chipotle mayo, combine mayonnaise, chipotle pepper, adobo sauce, and lime juice in a small bowl.
6. Toast the burger buns and assemble the burgers with the black bean patties, avocado slices, and a generous spread of chipotle mayo.
7. Serve immediately.

**Nutritional Facts:**

- Calories: 450
- Total Fat: 20g
- Total Carbs: 50g
- Fiber: 13g
- Net Carbs: 37g
- Protein: 15g

**Cooking Tip**: *For added texture and flavor in your black bean burgers, consider incorporating a small amount of finely chopped bell pepper or corn into the patty mixture. This not only adds color but also a subtle sweetness that complements the smoky spices.*

# Recipe 27: Tofu Scramble Tacos with Cilantro Lime Crema

*Prep Time: 20 mins - Cooking Time: 10 mins - Serves: 4*

**Ingredients:**

- 1 block (14 oz) firm tofu, drained and crumbled
- 1 tablespoon olive oil
- 1 small onion, diced
- 1 bell pepper, diced
- 1 teaspoon ground cumin
- 1/2 teaspoon chili powder
- 1/4 teaspoon turmeric (for color)
- Salt and pepper, to taste
- 8 small corn tortillas
- 1 cup fresh salsa

**For the Cilantro Lime Crema:**

- 1/2 cup sour cream (or vegan alternative)
- 1/4 cup fresh cilantro, chopped
- Juice and zest of 1 lime
- Salt, to taste

**Instructions:**

1. Heat olive oil in a pan over medium heat. Sauté onion and bell pepper until softened.
2. Add crumbled tofu to the pan. Stir in cumin, chili powder, turmeric, salt, and pepper. Cook for about 5-7 minutes, stirring frequently, until the tofu is heated through and begins to get a bit crispy.
3. While the tofu is cooking, prepare the cilantro lime crema. In a small bowl, mix together sour cream, cilantro, lime juice, and zest. Add salt to taste.
4. Warm the tortillas in a dry skillet or in the oven.
5. Assemble the tacos by placing a scoop of tofu scramble onto each tortilla. Top with fresh salsa.
6. Drizzle cilantro lime crema over the top of each taco.
7. Serve immediately and enjoy.

**Nutritional Facts:**

- Calories: 300
- Total Fat: 12g
- Total Carbs: 35g
- Fiber: 6g
- Net Carbs: 29g
- Protein: 15g

**Cooking Tip:** *For an extra boost of flavor, you can add a pinch of smoked paprika to the tofu scramble. It gives a smoky depth to the dish that pairs wonderfully with the freshness of the cilantro lime crema.*

# Recipe 28: Salmon with Roasted Brussels Sprouts and Balsamic Glaze

*Prep Time: 15 mins - Cooking Time: 25 mins - Serves: 4*

**Ingredients:**
- 4 salmon fillets (about 6 ounces each)
- 1 pound Brussels sprouts, halved
- 3 tablespoons olive oil, divided
- Salt and pepper, to taste
- 1/4 cup balsamic vinegar
- 2 tablespoons honey
- 1 clove garlic, minced

**Instructions:**
1. Preheat the oven to 400°F (200°C).
2. Toss the Brussels sprouts with 2 tablespoons of olive oil, salt, and pepper. Spread them on a baking sheet and roast for about 20 minutes or until tender and caramelized.
3. While the Brussels sprouts are roasting, prepare the balsamic glaze. In a small saucepan, combine balsamic vinegar, honey, and minced garlic. Bring to a simmer over medium heat and reduce until thickened about 5 minutes. Set aside.

4. Heat the remaining tablespoon of olive oil in a skillet over medium-high heat. Season the salmon fillets with salt and pepper. Please place them in the skillet, skin-side down, and cook for about 4 minutes. Flip and cook for another 3-4 minutes or until desired doneness.
5. To serve, place the salmon fillets on plates, accompanied by the roasted Brussels sprouts.
6. Drizzle the balsamic glaze over the salmon and Brussels sprouts.
7. Serve immediately, enjoying the combination of the savory salmon and the sweet, tangy glaze on the Brussels sprouts.

**Nutritional Facts:**
- Calories: 400
- Total Fat: 18g
- Total Carbs: 20g
- Fiber: 4g
- Net Carbs: 16g
- Protein: 35g

**Cooking Tip:** *For an added layer of flavor, sprinkle some lemon zest over the salmon before serving. The citrus aroma complements the richness of the salmon and the sweetness of the balsamic glaze.*

# Recipe 29: Turkey Meatloaf with Cranberry Glaze

*Prep Time: 20 mins - Cooking Time: 1 hr - Serves: 6*

## Ingredients:
- 2 pounds of ground turkey
- 1 onion, finely chopped
- 2 garlic cloves, minced
- 1 egg
- 1/2 cup breadcrumbs
- 1/4 cup milk
- 2 tablespoons Worcestershire sauce
- 1 teaspoon dried thyme
- 1 teaspoon dried sage
- Salt and pepper, to taste

## For the Cranberry Glaze:
- 1 cup cranberry sauce (canned or homemade)
- 2 tablespoons apple cider vinegar
- 2 tablespoons brown sugar
- 1/2 teaspoon ground mustard

## Instructions:
1. Preheat the oven to 350°F (175°C). Line a loaf pan with parchment paper or lightly grease it.
2. In a large bowl, combine the ground turkey, onion, garlic, egg, breadcrumbs, milk, Worcestershire sauce, thyme, sage, salt, and pepper. Mix until well combined, but do not overmix.
3. Press the meatloaf mixture into the prepared loaf pan.
4. In a small saucepan, combine cranberry sauce, apple cider vinegar, brown sugar, and ground mustard. Heat over medium, stirring until smooth and slightly reduced.
5. Spoon half of the cranberry glaze over the top of the meatloaf.
6. Bake the meatloaf for 45 minutes. Then, spoon the remaining cranberry glaze over the top and return to the oven for an additional 15 minutes or until the meatloaf is cooked through.
7. Let the meatloaf rest for 10 minutes before slicing.
8. Serve the meatloaf slices with any remaining glaze on the side.

## Nutritional Facts:
- Calories: 350
- Total Fat: 12g
- Total Carbs: 25g
- Fiber: 1g
- Net Carbs: 24g
- Protein: 35g

**Cooking Tip:** *Adding a grated apple to the meatloaf mixture can enhance the moisture and add a subtle sweetness that pairs nicely with the turkey and cranberry flavors.*

# Recipe 30: Vegetarian Chili with Quinoa and Black Beans

*Prep Time: 15 mins - Cooking Time: 40 mins - Serves: 6*

## Ingredients:

- 1 cup quinoa, rinsed
- 2 cans (15 oz each) black beans, drained and rinsed
- 1 large onion, chopped
- 2 bell peppers (any color), chopped
- 3 cloves garlic, minced
- 1 can (28 oz) crushed tomatoes
- 2 cups vegetable broth
- 1 tablespoon chili powder
- 1 teaspoon cumin
- 1 teaspoon smoked paprika
- 1/2 teaspoon cayenne pepper (optional for heat)
- Salt and pepper, to taste
- 2 tablespoons olive oil
- Optional toppings: avocado, sour cream, shredded cheese, cilantro, lime wedges

## Instructions:

1. Heat olive oil in a large pot over medium heat. Add onion and bell peppers, sautéing until softened.

2. Add garlic and sauté for another minute.

3. Stir in chili powder, cumin, smoked paprika, and cayenne pepper (if using). Cook for 2 minutes to allow the spices to become fragrant.

4. Add the quinoa, black beans, crushed tomatoes, and vegetable broth. Bring the mixture to a boil.

5. Reduce the heat to low, cover, and simmer for about 30 minutes, or until the quinoa is cooked and the chili has thickened.

6. Season with salt and pepper to taste.

7. Serve the chili hot, with optional toppings such as avocado, sour cream, shredded cheese, cilantro, or a squeeze of lime.

## Nutritional Facts:

- Calories: 320
- Total Fat: 7g
- Total Carbs: 52g
- Fiber: 14g
- Net Carbs: 38g
- Protein: 15g

**Cooking Tip:** *For an added depth of flavor, consider roasting the bell peppers before adding them to the chili. This brings out their natural sweetness and adds a smoky element to the dish.*

# Chapter 13: Delicious and Heart-Healthy Snack Recipes for Lower Cholesterol and Triglycerides

Welcome to a chapter where snacking is both a delight and a step towards better heart health. "10 Delicious and Heart-Healthy Snack Recipes for Lower Cholesterol and Triglycerides" is specially crafted for those who seek tasty yet healthy snack options. Understanding the importance of maintaining healthy cholesterol and triglyceride levels, this chapter is filled with recipes that are not only delicious but also beneficial for your heart.

Each snack recipe is designed with ingredients known for their heart-healthy properties. These snacks are perfect for those moments between meals when you crave something satisfying yet don't want to compromise on your health goals. From sweet treats to savory bites, these recipes offer a variety of flavors while focusing on nutrients that help manage cholesterol and triglyceride levels.

Dive into a collection of snack recipes that are as enjoyable as they are good for your heart. These snacks are easy to prepare, delicious, and perfect for keeping your cholesterol and triglycerides in check.

Each of these recipes is not just a treat for your taste buds but also a step towards a healthier heart. Whether you need a quick bite on the go or a relaxing treat at home, these snacks are your companions in maintaining a heart-healthy lifestyle without giving up the joy of snacking.

# Recipe 31: Veggie Sticks with Hummus and Edamame

*Prep Time: 15 mins - No Cooking - Serves: 4*

## Ingredients:

- 2 large carrots, peeled and cut into sticks
- 1 cucumber, cut into sticks
- 1 red bell pepper, cut into sticks
- 1 yellow bell pepper, cut into sticks
- 1 cup hummus (store-bought or homemade)
- 1 cup shelled edamame, cooked and cooled
- Optional: a pinch of sea salt or sesame seeds for the edamame

## Instructions:

1. Arrange the carrot, cucumber, and bell pepper sticks on a serving platter.

2. Place the hummus in a small bowl and set it on the platter alongside the vegetables.

3. In another small bowl, serve the cooked and cooled edamame. If desired, sprinkle the edamame with a pinch of sea salt or sesame seeds for extra flavor.

4. Enjoy the veggies by dipping them in the hummus and pair with a handful of edamame for added protein.

## Nutritional Facts:

- Calories (per serving): 180
- Total Fat: 9g
- Total Carbs: 20g
- Fiber: 6g
- Net Carbs: 14g
- Protein: 8g

**Cooking Tip:** *For a zesty twist, you can squeeze a bit of lemon juice over the veggie sticks or mix a little lemon zest into the hummus. This adds a refreshing citrus flavor that complements the creaminess of the hummus and the crunch of the vegetables.*

# Recipe 32: Baked Apple Chips with Cinnamon and Walnuts

*Prep Time: 10 mins - Cooking Time: 1 hr 30 mins - Serves: 4*

## Ingredients:

- 3 large apples (such as Fuji or Honeycrisp)
- 1 teaspoon ground cinnamon
- 1/2 cup walnuts, chopped

## Instructions:

1. Preheat the oven to 200°F (95°C). Line two baking sheets with parchment paper.

2. Core the apples and slice them very thinly, preferably with a mandoline slicer for uniform thickness.

3. Arrange the apple slices in a single layer on the prepared baking sheets.

4. Sprinkle the apple slices with ground cinnamon.

5. Bake in the preheated oven for about 1 hour and 30 minutes, flipping the apple slices halfway through the cooking time until they are dried out and crisp.

6. While the apples are baking, toast the chopped walnuts in a dry skillet over medium heat for about 3-5 minutes or until they are fragrant and slightly browned.

7. Once the apple chips are done, let them cool completely. They will crisp up more as they cool.

8. Sprinkle the toasted walnuts over the apple chips before serving.

## Nutritional Facts:

- Calories (per serving): 150
- Total Fat: 8g
- Total Carbs: 21g
- Fiber: 4g
- Net Carbs: 17g
- Protein: 2g

**Cooking Tip:** *For extra sweetness, you can lightly brush the apple slices with a small amount of maple syrup or honey before baking. This adds a lovely glaze and a deeper caramelized flavor to the apple chips.*

# Recipe 33: Air-fried chickpea Bites with Curry Spices

*Prep Time: 10 mins - Cooking Time: 15 mins - Serves: 4*

**Ingredients:**

- 2 cans (15 oz each) of chickpeas, drained, rinsed, and patted dry
- 2 tablespoons olive oil
- 1 teaspoon curry powder
- 1/2 teaspoon ground cumin
- 1/4 teaspoon ground turmeric
- 1/4 teaspoon paprika
- Salt and pepper, to taste

**Instructions:**

1. Preheat the air fryer to 390°F (200°C).

2. In a bowl, toss the chickpeas with olive oil, curry powder, cumin, turmeric, paprika, salt, and pepper until they are evenly coated.

3. Spread the chickpeas in an even layer in the air fryer basket. Avoid overcrowding, and cook in batches if necessary.

4. Air fry the chickpeas for 12-15 minutes, shaking the basket halfway through until they are golden brown and crispy.

5. Let the chickpeas cool slightly before serving. They will continue to crisp up as they cool.

**Nutritional Facts:**

- Calories (per serving): 210
- Total Fat: 8g
- Total Carbs: 28g
- Fiber: 8g
- Net Carbs: 20g
- Protein: 10g

**Cooking Tip:** *To keep the chickpeas crispy for longer, let them cool completely in the air fryer basket before transferring them to a container. This allows any residual moisture to evaporate and keeps them crunchy for snacking later.*

# Recipe 34: Yogurt Parfait with Berries and Chia Seeds

*Prep Time: 10 mins - No Cooking - Serves: 4*

## Ingredients:

- 2 cups plain yogurt (Greek or regular)
- 4 tablespoons chia seeds
- 2 cups mixed fresh berries (such as strawberries, blueberries, raspberries)
- 2 tablespoons honey or maple syrup (optional)
- 1/2 cup granola (optional)

## Instructions:

1. In a bowl, mix the yogurt with the chia seeds. If you prefer a little sweetness, stir in the honey or maple syrup.

2. Let the yogurt and chia mixture sit for about 5 minutes to allow the chia seeds to swell and thicken.

3. Start assembling the parfaits by spooning a layer of the yogurt mixture into 4 serving glasses or bowls.

4. Add a layer of mixed fresh berries over the yogurt.

5. Repeat the layers until all ingredients are used, finishing with a layer of berries on top.

6. If desired, top each parfait with a sprinkle of granola for added crunch.

7. Serve immediately or refrigerate for up to an hour before serving.

## Nutritional Facts:

- Calories (per serving): 180
- Total Fat: 5g
- Total Carbs: 28g
- Fiber: 6g
- Net Carbs: 22g
- Protein: 8g

**Cooking Tip:** *For an extra nutritional boost, sprinkle a pinch of ground cinnamon or a small handful of nuts like almonds or walnuts on top of the parfait. This adds not only a variety of textures but also contributes additional health benefits.*

# Recipe 35: Trail Mix with Nuts, Seeds, and Dried Fruit

*Prep Time: 10 mins - No Cooking - Serves: Varies*

## Ingredients:

- 1 cup almonds
- 1 cup walnuts
- 1/2 cup pumpkin seeds
- 1/2 cup sunflower seeds
- 1/2 cup dried cranberries
- 1/2 cup raisins
- Optional: 1/4 cup dark chocolate chips
- Optional: 1/4 cup coconut flakes
- Optional: a pinch of sea salt or a sprinkle of cinnamon for flavor

## Instructions:

1. In a large bowl, combine the almonds, walnuts, pumpkin seeds, and sunflower seeds.

2. Add the dried cranberries and raisins to the nut and seed mixture. Toss to combine evenly.

3. If using, add dark chocolate chips and coconut flakes to the mix. Stir gently to distribute.

-

4. If desired, season the trail mix with a pinch of sea salt or a sprinkle of cinnamon for an added flavor boost.

5. Once mixed, store the trail mix in an airtight container to maintain freshness.

6. Serve as a convenient and energy-boosting snack, perfect for on-the-go, hiking, or as a midday pick-me-up.

## Nutritional Facts (per serving, approximately 1/4 cup):

- Calories: 200
- Total Fat: 15g
- Total Carbs: 15g
- Fiber: 3g
- Net Carbs: 12g
- Protein: 5g

**Cooking Tip:** *Feel free to customize the trail mix based on your preferences or dietary needs. You can swap out any nuts or dried fruits for your favorites or add ingredients like banana chips, dried mango, or even a sprinkle of matcha powder for a unique twist.*

# Recipe 36: Roasted Seaweed Snacks with Sesame Oil

*Prep Time: 5 mins - Cooking Time: 10 mins - Serves: Varies*

## Ingredients:

- 10 sheets of nori (dried seaweed)
- 2 tablespoons sesame oil
- Sea salt, to taste
- Optional: a sprinkle of chili flakes or garlic powder for extra flavor

## Instructions:

1. Preheat the oven to 300°F (150°C). Line a baking sheet with parchment paper.

2. Lay the nori sheets on the baking sheet in a single layer. If they are too large, cut them into smaller, snack-sized pieces.

3. Lightly brush each nori sheet with sesame oil. Be sure to cover the entire surface, but don't saturate the seaweed.

4. Sprinkle a small amount of sea salt over the nori sheets. If using, add a sprinkle of chili flakes or garlic powder.

5. Place the baking sheet in the oven and roast the seaweed for 8-10 minutes. Keep a close eye on them to prevent burning.

6. The seaweed is ready when it turns a bit darker and crispy.

7. Remove from the oven and let the seaweed cool completely. It will continue to crisp up as it cools.

8. Once cooled, store the roasted seaweed snacks in an airtight container.

## Nutritional Facts (per serving, approximately 1 sheet):

- Calories: 20
- Total Fat: 2g
- Total Carbs: 1g
- Fiber: 1g
- Net Carbs: 0g
- Protein: 1g

**Cooking Tip:** *For a different flavor profile, try brushing the seaweed with a mixture of soy sauce and a drop of honey before roasting. This creates a sweet and savory glaze that enhances the natural umami flavor of the seaweed.*

# Recipe 37: Frozen Banana Bites with Dark Chocolate Dip

*Prep Time: 15 mins - Freezing Time: 2 hrs - Serves: 4*

## Ingredients:

- 4 ripe bananas
- 1 cup dark chocolate chips or chunks
- 1 tablespoon coconut oil
- Optional toppings: chopped nuts, shredded coconut, sea salt, or sprinkles

## Instructions:

1. Peel and slice the bananas into 1/2-inch thick rounds.

2. Arrange the banana slices on a baking sheet lined with parchment paper, ensuring they are not touching.

3. Freeze the banana slices for about 1 hour or until solid.

4. In a microwave-safe bowl, melt the dark chocolate with the coconut oil. Heat in 30-second intervals, stirring between each interval, until the chocolate is completely melted and smooth.

5. Dip each frozen banana slice into the melted chocolate, coating half or the entire slice as preferred.

6. Immediately sprinkle with any optional toppings like chopped nuts, shredded coconut, or a pinch of sea salt.

7. Place the chocolate-dipped banana bites back onto the parchment paper.

8. Freeze the banana bites for an additional hour or until the chocolate is set.

9. Once set, serve immediately or store in an airtight container in the freezer.

## Nutritional Facts (per serving, approximately 4 bites):

- Calories: 230
- Total Fat: 12g
- Total Carbs: 30g
- Fiber: 4g
- Net Carbs: 26g
- Protein: 3g

**Cooking Tip:** *To make this treat even more special, try drizzling the chocolate-dipped banana bites with a little bit of melted peanut butter or almond butter before the final freeze. This adds an extra layer of flavor and richness to the snack.*

# Recipe 38: Homemade Fruit and Vegetable Popsicles

*Prep Time: 20 mins - Freezing Time: 4 hrs - Serves: 6*

## Ingredients:
- 1 cup fresh spinach
- 1 banana, sliced
- 1 cup mixed berries (strawberries, blueberries, raspberries)
- 1/2 cup orange juice or apple juice
- 1/2 cup Greek yogurt or coconut yogurt (for a vegan option)
- 1 tablespoon honey or maple syrup (optional for added sweetness)

## Instructions:
1. In a blender, combine the spinach, banana, mixed berries, orange or apple juice, and yogurt. Blend until smooth.
2. Taste the mixture and add honey or maple syrup if you desire extra sweetness. Blend again to incorporate.
3. Pour the pureed mixture into popsicle molds, leaving a little space at the top as they will expand slightly when frozen.
4. Insert popsicle sticks into the molds. If the mixture is too soft to hold the sticks upright, freeze the popsicles for about 1 hour and then insert the sticks.
5. Freeze the popsicles for at least 4 hours or until completely solid.
6. To remove the popsicles from the molds, run the mold under warm water for a few seconds to loosen them.
7. Serve the popsicles immediately as a refreshing and healthy treat.

## Nutritional Facts (per popsicle):
- Calories: 60
- Total Fat: 0.5g
- Total Carbs: 12g
- Fiber: 2g
- Net Carbs: 10g
- Protein: 2g

**Cooking Tip:** *For a more layered effect, you can make these popsicles in two batches with different color blends. For instance, one batch with green veggies like spinach or kale and another with red or orange fruits. Pour one layer, freeze for an hour, then add the second layer and freeze again. This creates a visually appealing and nutritious treat.*

# Recipe 39: Cottage Cheese with Chopped Vegetables and Herbs

*Prep Time: 10 mins - No Cooking - Serves: 4*

## Ingredients:

- 2 cups cottage cheese
- 1 cucumber, finely diced
- 1 red bell pepper, finely diced
- 1/4 cup red onion, finely chopped
- 2 tablespoons fresh parsley, chopped
- 2 tablespoons fresh dill, chopped
- Salt and pepper, to taste
- Optional: a squeeze of lemon juice or a drizzle of olive oil for added flavor

## Instructions:

1. In a large bowl, combine the cottage cheese with the diced cucumber, red bell pepper, red onion, parsley, and dill.

2. Gently mix everything together until well combined.

3. Season the mixture with salt and pepper to taste. Add a squeeze of lemon juice or a drizzle of olive oil if desired for extra flavor.

4. Chill in the refrigerator for about 30 minutes to allow the flavors to meld together.

5. Serve the cottage cheese mixture as a refreshing and protein-packed snack or light lunch.

## Nutritional Facts (per serving):

- Calories: 130
- Total Fat: 2g
- Total Carbs: 10g
- Fiber: 1g
- Net Carbs: 9g
- Protein: 16g

**Cooking Tip:** *For a twist, add chopped tomatoes or avocado to the cottage cheese mixture. This not only adds more nutrients and flavors but also creates a more colorful and delicious dish.*

# Recipe 40: Edamame Hummus with Whole-Wheat Pita Chips

*Prep Time: 15 mins - Cooking Time: 10 mins (for pita chips) - Serves: 4*

## Ingredients:

- 2 cups shelled edamame, cooked and cooled
- 1/4 cup tahini
- 2 cloves garlic
- Juice of 1 lemon
- 2 tablespoons olive oil
- Salt and pepper, to taste
- 1/2 teaspoon ground cumin
- 3-4 tablespoons water, as needed for consistency

## For the Whole-Wheat Pita Chips:

- 4 whole-wheat pita breads
- 2 tablespoons olive oil
- Salt, to taste
- Optional: a sprinkle of garlic powder or paprika

## Instructions:

1. For the edamame hummus, place the cooked edamame, tahini, garlic, lemon juice, olive oil, salt, pepper, and cumin in a food processor.

2. Blend until smooth, adding water one tablespoon at a time until you reach your desired consistency.
3. Taste and adjust seasoning as needed.
4. Preheat the oven to 375°F (190°C).
5. Cut the pita bread into triangles and spread them out on a baking sheet.
6. Brush the pita triangles with olive oil and sprinkle with salt and optional garlic powder or paprika.
7. Bake the pita chips for 8-10 minutes or until they are crisp and golden.
8. Serve the edamame hummus with the whole-wheat pita chips.

## Nutritional Facts (per serving):

- Calories: 330
- Total Fat: 17g
- Total Carbs: 35g
- Fiber: 6g
- Net Carbs: 29g
- Protein: 15g

**Cooking Tip:** *For a zestier hummus, you can add a bit of grated lemon zest or a pinch of chili flakes for an extra kick. This will give the edamame hummus a refreshing twist and a slight heat that pairs well with the whole-wheat pita chips.*

# Chapter 14: Delicious and Heart-Healthy Side Dishes to Round Out Your Meals:

Welcome to a chapter dedicated to enriching your meals with both flavor and health. In "10 Delicious and Heart-Healthy Side Dishes to Round Out Your Meals," we dive into a world where taste and well-being go hand in hand. This chapter is designed for anyone looking to add a nutritious touch to their dining table without sacrificing the joy of a delicious meal.

Heart health is a crucial aspect of overall well-being, and the foods we choose to put on our plates play a significant role. These recipes are crafted not only with the intention of tantalizing your taste buds but also to support a heart-healthy lifestyle. From the crunch of fresh vegetables to the richness of wholesome grains, each recipe is a celebration of ingredients that are both nourishing and satisfying.

In this chapter, you'll discover a collection of side dishes that are as good for your heart as they are for your palate. We've carefully selected a variety of recipes that cater to diverse tastes and dietary needs, ensuring there's something for everyone.

Each recipe in this chapter not only contributes to a heart-healthy diet but also ensures that your meals are a delightful experience. Whether you're looking for a quick and easy side or something a bit more elaborate, these dishes are sure to become staples in your culinary repertoire.

# Recipe 41: Roasted Brussels Sprouts with Balsamic Glaze and Pecans

*Prep Time: 10 mins - Cooking Time: 25 mins - Serves: 4*

## Ingredients:

- 1 pound Brussels sprouts, trimmed and halved
- 2 tablespoons olive oil
- Salt and pepper, to taste
- 1/4 cup balsamic vinegar
- 2 tablespoons brown sugar
- 1/2 cup pecans, roughly chopped

## Instructions:

1. Preheat the oven to 400°F (200°C).

2. Toss the Brussels sprouts with olive oil, salt, and pepper. Spread them out in a single layer on a baking sheet.

3. Roast in the preheated oven for 20-25 minutes or until the Brussels sprouts are crispy on the outside and tender on the inside.

4. While the Brussels sprouts are roasting, prepare the balsamic glaze.

In a small saucepan, combine the balsamic vinegar and brown sugar. Bring to a simmer over medium heat and reduce until the mixture thickens into a glaze, about 5-7 minutes.

5. Once the Brussels sprouts are done, transfer them to a serving dish.

6. Drizzle the balsamic glaze over the roasted Brussels sprouts.

7. Sprinkle the chopped pecans on top.

8. Serve immediately as a delicious and flavorful side dish.

## Nutritional Facts (per serving):

- Calories: 220
- Total Fat: 15g
- Total Carbs: 20g
- Fiber: 4g
- Net Carbs: 16g
- Protein: 4g

**Cooking Tip:** *For an extra burst of flavor, you can add a sprinkle of grated Parmesan cheese over the Brussels sprouts after adding the balsamic glaze and pecans. This adds a savory and cheesy dimension to the dish.*

# Recipe 42: Quinoa Pilaf with Lemon and Herbs

*Prep Time: 10 mins - Cooking Time: 20 mins - Serves: 4*

## Ingredients:

- 1 cup quinoa, rinsed and drained
- 2 cups vegetable broth or water
- 1 tablespoon olive oil
- 1 small onion, finely chopped
- 2 cloves garlic, minced
- Zest and juice of 1 lemon
- 1/4 cup fresh parsley, chopped
- 1/4 cup fresh basil, chopped
- Salt and pepper, to taste

## Instructions:

1. Heat olive oil in a saucepan over medium heat. Add the onion and garlic, sautéing until the onion is translucent, about 5 minutes.

2. Add the rinsed quinoa to the saucepan and cook for 1-2 minutes, stirring frequently.

3. Pour in the vegetable broth or water and bring to a boil.

4. Reduce the heat to low, cover the saucepan, and simmer for about 15 minutes, or until all the liquid is absorbed and the quinoa is fluffy.

5. Remove the saucepan from the heat. Stir in the lemon zest, lemon juice, parsley, and basil. Season with salt and pepper to taste.

6. Fluff the quinoa with a fork and serve as a nutritious and flavorful side dish.

## Nutritional Facts (per serving):

- Calories: 220
- Total Fat: 5g
- Total Carbs: 35g
- Fiber: 4g
- Net Carbs: 31g
- Protein: 8g

**Cooking Tip:** *To enhance the nutty flavor of quinoa, you can toast the grains in the saucepan for a few minutes before adding the liquid. This adds depth to the pilaf and brings out the quinoa's natural flavors.*

# Recipe 43: Roasted Butternut Squash with Honey and Sage

*Prep Time: 15 mins - Cooking Time: 30 mins - Serves: 4*

### Ingredients:

- 1 medium butternut squash, peeled, seeded, and cut into wedges
- 2 tablespoons olive oil
- 2 tablespoons honey
- 1/4 cup fresh sage leaves, finely chopped
- 1/2 teaspoon ground cinnamon
- Salt and pepper, to taste

### Instructions:

1. Preheat the oven to 400°F (200°C).

2. In a large bowl, toss the butternut squash wedges with olive oil, honey, chopped sage, cinnamon, salt, and pepper until well coated.

3. Spread the squash wedges in a single layer on a baking sheet lined with parchment paper.

4. Roast in the preheated oven for about 30 minutes, or until the squash is tender and the edges are caramelized, flipping the wedges halfway through the cooking time.

5. Remove from the oven and let cool slightly.

6. Serve the roasted butternut squash as a delicious and aromatic side dish, perfect for fall and winter meals.

### Nutritional Facts (per serving):

- Calories: 180
- Total Fat: 7g
- Total Carbs: 30g
- Fiber: 3g
- Net Carbs: 27g
- Protein: 2g

**Cooking Tip:** *For an extra burst of flavor, you can sprinkle a little bit of grated Parmesan cheese or crumbled feta over the roasted squash just before serving. This adds a savory element that complements the sweetness of the honey and the warmth of the cinnamon.*

# Recipe 44: Grilled Portobello Mushrooms with Balsamic Vinaigrette

*Prep Time: 20 mins (including marination) - Cooking Time: 10 mins - Serves: 4*

**Ingredients:**
- 4 large portobello mushrooms, stems removed
- 1/4 cup balsamic vinegar
- 1/4 cup olive oil
- 2 cloves garlic, minced
- 1 teaspoon dried thyme
- Salt and pepper, to taste

**For the Balsamic Vinaigrette:**
- 1/4 cup balsamic vinegar
- 1/2 cup olive oil
- 1 teaspoon Dijon mustard
- 1 teaspoon honey
- Salt and pepper, to taste

**Instructions:**
1. In a small bowl, whisk together 1/4 cup balsamic vinegar, 1/4 cup olive oil, minced garlic, thyme, salt, and pepper.
2. Place the portobello mushrooms in a shallow dish and pour the marinade over them. Ensure the mushrooms are well coated. Let them marinate for 15 minutes.
3. Preheat the grill to medium-high heat.
4. Grill the marinated mushrooms for about 5 minutes on each side or until they are tender and have grill marks.
5. While the mushrooms are grilling, prepare the balsamic vinaigrette. In a bowl, whisk together 1/4 cup balsamic vinegar, 1/2 cup olive oil, Dijon mustard, honey, salt, and pepper until emulsified.
6. Once the mushrooms are done, transfer them to a serving platter.
7. Drizzle the balsamic vinaigrette over the grilled mushrooms.
8. Serve the grilled portobello mushrooms as a hearty and flavorful side dish.

**Nutritional Facts (per serving):**
- Calories: 300
- Total Fat: 27g
- Total Carbs: 10g
- Fiber: 1g
- Net Carbs: 9g
- Protein: 2g

**Cooking Tip**: *For an added layer of flavor, you can sprinkle some freshly grated Parmesan cheese or crumbled goat cheese over the mushrooms just before serving. The cheese adds a creamy texture and a savory depth to the dish.*

# Recipe 45: Green Beans with Garlic and Toasted Almonds

*Prep Time: 10 mins - Cooking Time: 15 mins - Serves: 4*

## Ingredients:

- 1 pound green beans, trimmed
- 2 tablespoons olive oil
- 3 cloves garlic, minced
- 1/2 cup almonds, sliced
- Salt and pepper, to taste

## Instructions:

1. Bring a large pot of salted water to a boil. Add the green beans and cook for 3-5 minutes or until they are tender but still crisp. Drain and set aside.

2. In a dry skillet, toast the sliced almonds over medium heat, stirring frequently, until they are golden and fragrant. Remove from the skillet and set aside.

3. In the same skillet, heat the olive oil over medium heat. Add the minced garlic and sauté for about 1 minute, or until it is fragrant but not browned.

4. Add the cooked green beans to the skillet with the garlic. Toss to coat the beans in the garlic and oil. Season with salt and pepper.

5. Cook for another 2-3 minutes, stirring occasionally, until the green beans are heated through.

6. Transfer the green beans to a serving dish and sprinkle the toasted almonds over the top.

7. Serve the green beans warm as a flavorful and nutritious side dish.

## Nutritional Facts (per serving):

- Calories: 180
- Total Fat: 14g
- Total Carbs: 10g
- Fiber: 4g
- Net Carbs: 6g
- Protein: 5g

**Cooking Tip:** *For a zesty twist, add a squeeze of fresh lemon juice over the green beans just before serving. The lemon juice adds a bright, fresh flavor that pairs perfectly with the garlic and almonds.*

# Recipe 46: Lentil Salad with Cucumber, Tomato, and Feta

*Prep Time: 15 mins - No Cooking (if using pre-cooked lentils) - Serves: 4*

## Ingredients:

- 2 cups cooked lentils (green or brown)
- 1 large cucumber, diced
- 2 tomatoes, diced
- 1/2 cup feta cheese, crumbled
- 1/4 cup red onion, finely chopped
- 1/4 cup fresh parsley, chopped
- 3 tablespoons olive oil
- Juice of 1 lemon
- Salt and pepper, to taste

## Instructions:

1. In a large bowl, combine the cooked lentils, diced cucumber, diced tomatoes, crumbled feta cheese, red onion, and chopped parsley.

2. In a small bowl, whisk together the olive oil, lemon juice, salt, and pepper to create the vinaigrette.

3. Pour the vinaigrette over the lentil mixture and gently toss to combine, ensuring the salad is evenly coated.

4. Season the salad with additional salt and pepper to taste.

5. Let the salad chill in the refrigerator for at least 30 minutes to allow the flavors to meld.

6. Serve the lentil salad as a refreshing and protein-rich side dish or a light meal.

## Nutritional Facts (per serving):

- Calories: 250
- Total Fat: 12g
- Total Carbs: 26g
- Fiber: 10g
- Net Carbs: 16g
- Protein: 12g

**Cooking Tip:** For an added crunch, you can include some chopped bell peppers or celery in the salad. Additionally, a sprinkle of fresh mint or dill can provide a fresh and aromatic touch to the dish.

# Recipe 47: Roasted Sweet Potato Mash with Maple Pecan Crumble

*Prep Time: 15 mins - Cooking Time: 40 mins - Serves: 4*

**Ingredients:**
- 4 large sweet potatoes, peeled and cubed
- 2 tablespoons butter (or vegan alternative)
- 2 tablespoons maple syrup
- Salt and pepper, to taste

**For the Maple Pecan Crumble:**
- 1/2 cup pecans, chopped
- 1/4 cup rolled oats
- 2 tablespoons flour (can use gluten-free)
- 2 tablespoons brown sugar
- 2 tablespoons melted butter (or vegan alternative)
- 1/2 teaspoon cinnamon

**Instructions:**
1. Preheat the oven to 400°F (200°C).
2. Spread the sweet potato cubes on a baking sheet. Roast for about 30-35 minutes or until tender and slightly caramelized.
3. While the sweet potatoes are roasting, prepare the maple pecan crumble. In a bowl, combine the chopped pecans, rolled oats, flour, brown sugar, melted butter, and cinnamon. Mix until well combined.
4. Spread the crumble mixture on a small baking sheet and bake in the oven alongside the sweet potatoes for 10-15 minutes or until golden and crispy.
5. Once the sweet potatoes are done, remove them from the oven and mash them with butter and maple syrup. Season with salt and pepper.
6. Transfer the mashed sweet potatoes to a serving dish. Top with the maple pecan crumble.
7. Serve warm as a delicious and comforting side dish.

**Nutritional Facts (per serving):**
- Calories: 320
- Total Fat: 15g
- Total Carbs: 45g
- Fiber: 6g
- Net Carbs: 39g
- Protein: 4g

**Cooking Tip:** *For an extra layer of flavor, you can add a pinch of nutmeg or ginger to the sweet potato mash. These spices complement the natural sweetness of the potatoes and the richness of the maple pecan crumble.*

# Recipe 48: Sautéed Kale with Garlic and Lemon

*Prep Time: 10 mins - Cooking Time: 10 mins - Serves: 4*

## Ingredients:

- 2 bunches kale, stems removed and leaves chopped
- 2 tablespoons olive oil
- 3 cloves garlic, minced
- Juice of 1 lemon
- Salt and pepper, to taste
- Optional: red pepper flakes for heat

## Instructions:

1. Heat the olive oil in a large skillet over medium heat.

2. Add the minced garlic to the skillet and sauté for about 1 minute or until fragrant but not browned.

3. Add the chopped kale to the skillet. Sauté, frequently stirring, until the kale begins to wilt and becomes tender about 5-7 minutes.

4. Squeeze the lemon juice over the kale and toss to combine. Season with salt and pepper to taste. If using, sprinkle some red pepper flakes for a bit of heat.

5. Serve the sautéed kale immediately as a nutrient-rich and flavorful side dish.

## Nutritional Facts (per serving):

- Calories: 100
- Total Fat: 7g
- Total Carbs: 10g
- Fiber: 2g
- Net Carbs: 8g
- Protein: 3g

**Cooking Tip:** *To add a bit of crunch and nuttiness to the dish, you can sprinkle toasted pine nuts or sliced almonds over the kale just before serving. This not only adds texture but also enriches the overall flavor profile of the dish.*

# Recipe 49: Couscous Salad with Roasted Vegetables and Herbs

*Prep Time: 20 mins - Cooking Time: 30 mins - Serves: 4*

**Ingredients:**

- 1 cup couscous
- 1 zucchini, chopped
- 1 red bell pepper, chopped
- 1 yellow bell pepper, chopped
- 1 red onion, chopped
- 2 tablespoons olive oil
- Salt and pepper, to taste
- 1/4 cup fresh parsley, chopped
- 1/4 cup fresh basil, chopped
- 1/4 cup fresh mint, chopped

**For the Vinaigrette:**

- 1/4 cup olive oil
- 2 tablespoons red wine vinegar
- 1 garlic clove, minced
- 1 teaspoon Dijon mustard
- Salt and pepper, to taste

**Instructions:**

1. Preheat the oven to 400°F (200°C).
2. Spread the chopped zucchini, bell peppers, and red onion on a baking sheet. Drizzle with 2 tablespoons of olive oil and season with salt and pepper. Toss to coat evenly.
3. Roast the vegetables in the oven for about 25-30 minutes or until tender and slightly caramelized.
4. While the vegetables are roasting, prepare the couscous according to package instructions.
5. In a small bowl, whisk together the ingredients for the vinaigrette: olive oil, red wine vinegar, minced garlic, Dijon mustard, salt, and pepper.
6. In a large bowl, combine the cooked couscous, roasted vegetables, chopped parsley, basil, and mint.
7. Drizzle the vinaigrette over the salad and toss to combine everything evenly.
8. Season with additional salt and pepper if needed.
9. Serve the couscous salad as a bright and flavorful side dish.

**Nutritional Facts (per serving):**

- Calories: 350
- Total Fat: 15g
- Total Carbs: 45g
- Fiber: 5g
- Net Carbs: 40g
- Protein: 8g

**Cooking Tip:** *For an extra burst of flavor, add a squeeze of fresh lemon juice or a handful of crumbled feta cheese to the salad before serving. These additions provide a refreshing tang and a creamy texture, enhancing the overall taste of the salad.*

# Recipe 50: Grilled Asparagus with Parmesan and Lemon

*Prep Time: 10 mins - Cooking Time: 10 mins - Serves: 4*

## Ingredients:

- 1 pound asparagus, ends trimmed
- 2 tablespoons olive oil
- Salt and pepper, to taste
- Juice of 1 lemon
- 1/4 cup Parmesan cheese, grated
- Lemon wedges for serving

## Instructions:

1. Preheat your grill to medium-high heat.

2. Toss the asparagus stalks with olive oil and season with salt and pepper.

3. Grill the asparagus for about 4-5 minutes on each side or until they are tender and slightly charred.

4. Once grilled, transfer the asparagus to a serving platter.

5. Squeeze fresh lemon juice over the grilled asparagus.

6. Sprinkle the grated Parmesan cheese evenly over the top.

7. Serve the grilled asparagus immediately, accompanied by additional lemon wedges.

## Nutritional Facts (per serving):

- Calories: 120
- Total Fat: 9g
- Total Carbs: 6g
- Fiber: 3g
- Net Carbs: 3g
- Protein: 5g

**Cooking Tip:** *For an extra touch of elegance, you can garnish the asparagus with some lemon zest or a few thinly sliced almonds. This not only adds a beautiful presentation but also introduces additional flavors and textures to the dish.*

# Chapter 15: Bonus Section Based On A Holistic Approach

Welcome to Chapter 15, a special bonus section that embraces a holistic approach to health and well-being. This chapter is a unique addition, offering insights and practices that go beyond traditional recipes and dietary advice. It's designed for those who recognize that true health encompasses not just what we eat but also how we live, think, and interact with our environment.

In this chapter, you'll find a diverse range of content that touches upon various aspects of a holistic lifestyle. From mindfulness practices and stress management techniques to physical exercises and environmental considerations, each topic is chosen with the aim of enhancing overall well-being.

Dive into a comprehensive guide that integrates multiple dimensions of health and wellness:

This chapter is a treasure trove of information and practices that offer a comprehensive view of health. It's designed to inspire and guide you in your journey towards a more balanced, healthy, and fulfilled life, acknowledging that every aspect of our daily lives contributes to our overall well-being.

# Bonus Chapter 15.1: Mind-Body Connection in Health

## Understanding the Connection between Body and Mind

Embarking on a journey towards health requires us to acknowledge the link between our mental and physical well-being. In this chapter, we delve into the ways in which our thoughts, emotions, and mental state directly impact our health, with a particular focus on cholesterol levels and heart health. Contemporary research consistently demonstrates that stress, anxiety, and other psychological factors can have effects on our bodies and our cardiovascular system.

## The Influence of Stress on Cholesterol Levels

Chronic stress plays a role in altering cholesterol levels. When we experience stress, our bodies release cortisol and adrenaline. Hormones that initiate a "fight or flight" response. While this response can be beneficial in bursts, prolonged exposure to stress can lead to high cholesterol levels. High levels of cortisol can stimulate the liver to produce cholesterol, resulting in an imbalance that increases the risk of heart disease.

## Techniques for Managing Stress

**1. Mindfulness and Meditation:** These practices involve focusing on the moment and acknowledging one's thoughts and feelings without judgment. Regular engagement in mindfulness and meditation can effectively reduce stress levels while also lowering cortisol levels.

**2. Breathing Exercises:** Simple yet controlled breathing techniques help calm the mind and alleviate stress.

Incorporating techniques, like breathing or pranayama, into our routines can be quite effortless.

**3. Regular Exercise:** Engaging in activity is beneficial not only for our bodies but also for our minds. It triggers the release of endorphins, which are natural mood boosters that aid in reducing stress levels.

**4. Sufficient Sleep:** Getting quality sleep is crucial for maintaining health. Establishing a sleep schedule can significantly minimize stress and its adverse effects on our well-being.

## The Power of Positive Thinking

Having a positive outlook can profoundly impact our health. Positive thinking helps us cope with stress and often results in making lifestyle choices. Research indicates that individuals with an attitude typically have cholesterol levels, possibly due to better stress management and overall healthier habits.

## Cultivating a Balanced Lifestyle

Maintaining a lifestyle is fundamental to achieving health. This entails not only taking care of our well-being through proper diet and exercise but also nurturing our mental and emotional wellness. Activities such as yoga, tai chi, or spending time in nature can contribute to finding this equilibrium. Moreover, building connections and engaging in hobbies play significant roles in promoting mental well-being.

---

*Recognizing the connection between mind and body is essential for wellness.*

---

By recognizing and utilizing this link, people can greatly enhance their heart health and cholesterol levels. This section emphasizes the significance of well-being in the pursuit of health and long life, urging readers to embrace practices that nurture both their minds and bodies.

The purpose of this chapter is to offer a comprehension of how mental health influences physical well-being, particularly in relation to cholesterol and heart health. It provides guidance on stress management. Fostering a positive outlook is a crucial element in the quest for optimal health.

# Bonus Chapter 15.2: The Power of Sleep and Rest

### Understanding the Importance of Sleep

Ssleep goes beyond being a period of rest. It is an aspect of our overall health and well-being. In this chapter, we delve into the role that sleep plays in maintaining health. Specifically, we explore how it regulates cholesterol and triglyceride levels while enhancing metabolic functions. Quality sleep is just as crucial as having a diet and engaging in exercise when it comes to achieving optimal health.

### The Connection between Sleep and Cholesterol

Recent studies have revealed a correlation between sleep patterns and cholesterol levels. When we experience sleep or irregular sleeping habits, it can disrupt our body's metabolic processes, including how it processes and utilizes cholesterol. This disruption can lead to elevated LDL ( cholesterol) levels. Decreased HDL (good cholesterol) levels, thereby increasing the risk of heart disease.

### Metabolic Benefits Derived from Quality Sleep

Ensuring sleep is vital for our bodies' metabolic health. While we sleep, our bodies perform functions such as regulating hormones that control appetite, stress responses, and energy utilization. By obtaining quality sleep, we help maintain a balance of these hormones, which aids in weight management and reduces the likelihood of developing metabolic disorders.

## Effective Strategies for Promoting Restful Sleep

- Developing a consistent sleep routine Going to bed and waking up at the time every day is beneficial for regulating our body clock, which ultimately results in better sleep quality.

- Creating a tranquil sleeping environment: A lit and comfortably cool atmosphere can greatly enhance the quality of our sleep. Investing in a mattress and pillows can also make a difference.

- Reducing screen exposure before bedtime The blue light emitted by screens can disrupt the production of melatonin, which is responsible for regulating our sleep. To promote sleep, it's advisable to limit screen time leading up to bedtime.

- Engaging in relaxation techniques Activities like reading, taking a bath, or gently stretching before bed can help relax the body and prepare it for sleep.

- Being mindful of what we consume and avoiding meals, caffeine, and alcohol at bedtime can positively impact our ability to achieve restful sleep.

## Recognizing the importance of maintaining sleep patterns

Consistency plays a role when it comes to achieving restorative sleep. Irregular sleeping patterns can disrupt our rhythms, leading to compromised sleep quality and potential negative effects on our overall health.

## Addressing sleep disorders

Sleep disorders such as insomnia, sleep apnea, and restless leg syndrome have implications for our well-being. It's crucial to seek attention and treatment if experiencing any of these conditions.

It's crucial to prioritize seeking assistance and appropriate treatment for these conditions as it greatly contributes to maintaining health and well-being.

## In conclusion

Recognizing the significance of sleep and rest is vital when aiming for health. Getting quality sleep plays a role in managing cholesterol, metabolic health, and overall well-being. By adopting sleep habits and addressing any sleep disorders, individuals can take a step towards leading a healthier life.

This chapter highlights the role of sleep in promoting health, specifically in regulating cholesterol and triglyceride levels. It offers strategies to achieve sleep while emphasizing the importance of addressing any existing sleep disorders. The key message is clear: making sleep a priority is essential for anyone striving to improve their health and increase longevity.

# Bonus Chapter 15.3: Holistic Nutrition Beyond Cholesterol

## Understanding Holistic Nutrition

Holistic nutrition focuses on nourishing the body, mind, and spirit through the food we consume. It goes beyond managing cholesterol levels. Instead, it embraces a dietary approach that promotes overall well-being. This chapter aims to provide a perspective on diet, shedding light on how maintaining a diet and practicing mindful eating can significantly contribute to longevity and overall health.

## The Significance of a Well-Balanced Diet

A balanced diet lies at the core of nutrition. It involves incorporating a range of foods that offer the nutrients required for optimal bodily functions. This includes

- Fruits and Vegetables These are packed with vitamins, minerals, and antioxidants.
- Whole Grains provide fiber for digestion and ample energy.
- Lean Proteins are Essential for muscle growth and repair.
- Healthy Fats Necessary for hormone production and maintaining cellular health.

## Adopting Mindful Eating Habits

Eating revolves around being fully present during meals, savoring each bite, and being attuned to your body's hunger and fullness signals. Practicing eating can help prevent overeating, improve digestion, and enhance one's appreciation for food. Quality matters as much as quantity.

## Gut Health's Influence on Overall Well-being

The gut is often referred to as the " brain" because it has an impact on our overall health and well-being. A healthy gut not only contributes to an immune system but also improves heart health, brain function, mood, sleep quality, and digestion. Including probiotics and prebiotics in our diet can help support the health of our gut.

## Nutrients for a Long and Healthy Life

- Nutrients play roles in promoting longevity and overall wellness

- Antioxidants fight against oxidative stress and lower the risk of chronic diseases.

- Omega 3 Fatty Acids These are essential for maintaining heart health and cognitive functions.

- Fiber plays a role in supporting health and regulating blood sugar levels.

- Vitamins and Minerals Each vitamin and mineral has its own specific role, from boosting immune function to promoting strong bones.

## Adapting Our Diet to Different Life Stages

As we go through stages of life, our dietary needs change accordingly. This section will discuss how nutritional requirements vary across life stages and provide guidance on adjusting your diet to ensure health.

## In Conclusion

Holistic nutrition encompasses an approach to eating and living that goes beyond managing cholesterol levels. It emphasizes nourishing every aspect of our being for long-term health and well-being.

By adopting a rounded eating plan, being mindful of our food choices, giving importance to the health of our gut, and having knowledge about the role different nutrients play, we can greatly improve our well-being and quality of life.

This chapter provides an examination of nutrition, emphasizing the significance of maintaining balance and mindfulness when it comes to eating. It highlights the role that gut health plays and how various nutrients impact our wellness. Readers are given a guide to follow for a nourishing lifestyle that promotes long-term health and vitality.

# Bonus Chapter 15.4: Integrative Approaches to Health

### Exploring an Integrated Approach to Health

Integrative health is an approach that combines medical practices with alternative and complementary therapies to promote overall well-being. In this chapter, we will delve into the management of cholesterol and the promotion of heart health through the integration of health modalities. It is essential to note that consulting with healthcare professionals remains crucial throughout this process.

### The Significance of Herbal Remedies

For centuries, herbal remedies have been utilized to address health concerns, including heart health and cholesterol management. Garlic, turmeric, and ginger are herbs known for their inflammatory properties and ability to lower cholesterol levels. This section will guide you on how to incorporate these remedies into your daily routine.

### Acupuncture Impact on Heart Health

Acupuncture forms a part of Chinese medicine by utilizing fine needles inserted at specific points on the body to rebalance energy flow. Research suggests that acupuncture can effectively reduce blood pressure, alleviate stress, and enhance heart health. In this chapter segment, we will explore the mechanisms behind acupunctures' effectiveness. Provide insights into what you can expect during a session.

## Other Complementary Therapies

In addition to remedies and acupuncture, various complementary therapies can contribute to supporting heart health:

- Yoga and Tai Chi These practices encompass postures, breathing exercises, and meditation techniques that help reduce stress levels while improving cardiovascular well-being.

- Massage TherapyRegular massages have been shown to have an impact on reducing stress and anxiety, both of which can contribute to cholesterol levels and heart disease.

- Aromatherapy using oils can help promote relaxation and alleviate stress, ultimately benefiting heart health.

## The Importance of Finding Balance

While alternative therapies like these can be beneficial, it's important to remember that they should be used as treatments alongside medical care. Striking a balance between these approaches is crucial for effectively addressing all aspects of health.

## Seeking Guidance from Healthcare Professionals

Before incorporating any therapy into your routine, it's essential to consult with healthcare professionals who can provide guidance. They will consider your health needs and medical history to help you integrate these practices effectively into your health plan.

## In Conclusion

Integrative approaches offer a way to manage cholesterol levels and foster heart health. By combining treatments with alternative therapies, individuals can take a more holistic approach to their well-being. This chapter aims to shed light on practices while emphasizing the significance of seeking professional advice when adopting these methods for optimal health.

This chapter delves into the integration of medicine with alternative healing practices to create a well-rounded approach toward achieving overall wellness. The content includes subjects such as remedies and acupuncture, consistently emphasizing the importance of consulting professionals to ensure safe and efficient health management.

# Bonus Chapter 15.5: Building Sustainable Health Habits

Embarking on a journey towards health is not a quick race but rather a steady marathon. The final chapter of this guide focuses on transforming short-term health adjustments into sustainable habits. Key elements in this transformative process involve understanding the psychology behind habit formation, setting goals, and creating an environment that nurtures these habits.

### Understanding the Psychology of Habit Formation

Habit formation runs in our makeup. It involves the development of behaviors that become natural over time. This section delves into how habits shape the role of cues and rewards and the significance of consistency. By grasping these principles, you can deliberately design habits that truly stick.

### Setting Goals

Establishing attainable goals is crucial when striving for sustainable health habits. These goals should adhere to the SMART criteria: Specific, Measurable, Achievable, Relevant, and Time-bound. In this chapter, you'll be guided on how to set goals and break them down into steps that are more manageable and, thus, easier to achieve.

## Creating a Supportive Environment

Your environment plays a role in shaping your habits. This encompasses both your surroundings and your social circles. Building an environment that supports your health aspirations can significantly bolster your chances of success. This could involve stocking up on foods, becoming a member of a fitness group, or even involving your family and friends in your journey towards health.

## Real-Life Success Stories

Stories of individuals who have successfully transformed their lifestyles serve as an inspiration. Provide insights. These real-life examples showcase strategies and approaches that have proven effective in offering encouragement and guidance to readers.

## Overcoming Common Challenges

Change doesn't come without its share of obstacles. This section addresses challenges such as lack of time, motivation, and setbacks. It provides strategies for overcoming these hurdles while highlighting the importance of resilience and adaptability throughout the health journey.

## Integrating Healthy Habits into Everyday Life

The ultimate goal is to incorporate these habits into your daily routine. This means making them as natural as any activity. The chapter will provide tips on how to integrate these habits into your life.

## Conclusion

Developing health habits is a process that requires patience, dedication, and a strategic approach. This chapter equips you with the knowledge and tools needed to transform short-term changes into habits, putting you on a path toward a healthier and more fulfilling life.

In this chapter, you'll find a handbook on how to develop lasting healthy habits. It delves into the psychology behind forming habits, setting goals, and creating an environment. Through examples and practical tips, it seeks to motivate and aid readers in making changes for a healthier future.

# Chapter 16: Conclusion

In this book, we have delved into the captivating realm of health and longevity, exploring the secrets to achieving well-being. Our journey has covered aspects of our lives, including nutrition, exercise, mindset, and lifestyle choices. The ultimate aim has been to attain a vibrant life. As we come to the end of this expedition, let us recap the lessons and main points that have been discussed.

**The Importance of Nutrition:** We've discovered how crucial it is to nourish our bodies with foods packed with nutrients. A balanced diet that includes plenty of fruits, vegetables, lean proteins, and whole grains serves as a foundation for good health and longevity. By prioritizing foods and limiting our consumption of added sugars, unhealthy fats, and processed foods, we unlock our body's potential to thrive.

**The Significance of Physical Activity:** Regular exercise is not only vital for maintaining weight but also for strengthening our bodies and improving overall well-being. Engaging in a mix of exercises, strength training sessions, and flexibility workouts can enhance health while boosting our immune systems and sharpening mental clarity.

*It's important to keep in mind that even small amounts of activity can have an impact on our health.*

**The Role of Mental and Emotional Well-Being:** Our mental and emotional well-being plays a role in our health. Chronic stress, emotions and harmful thought patterns can deeply affect our well-being. By practicing mindfulness, managing stress effectively, and nurturing relationships, we can build a foundation for optimal health and longevity.

**Importance of Sleep and Rest:** Getting sleep is vital for our bodies to repair, regenerate, and function at their best. Prioritizing quality sleep and creating a sleep environment can enhance function, improve mood, and help prevent various chronic diseases. Remember to establish a consistent sleep routine and incorporate relaxation techniques to improve both the quality and duration of your sleep.

**The Impact of Lifestyle Choices:** Our habits and lifestyle choices have the power to shape the trajectory of our health. By avoiding smoking, limiting alcohol consumption, and reducing exposure to toxins, we can protect our bodies against various diseases. Additionally, incorporating stress management techniques into our lives, cultivating relationships, and finding purpose can contribute to our well-being.

As you begin your quest for health and long life, I want to share some motivating words. Keep in mind that this is a journey and every effort you make to enhance your well-being counts. Embrace the knowledge you gain from this book and apply it to your life. Remember, the power to shape your future lies in your hands when it comes to your health and longevity.

During moments of uncertainty or challenges, remind yourself of the individuals who have turned their lives around and achieved levels of health. Take inspiration from their stories. Believe that you, too, can make a difference. It may not always be sailing. The rewards outweigh the obstacles.

Surround yourself with a supportive community of like-minded individuals who share your passion for well-being and a long life. Seek mentors who can guide you on this journey. Remember that you're not alone in striving for health and longevity—we are all working towards the goal.

*Never underestimate the impact of changes. It's through these steps that significant transformations occur.*

Please make a commitment to incorporate one positive change into your daily life, no matter how small it may seem. Whether it is opting for a meal or taking some time out for self-care, each choice you make will have an effect and contribute to your overall well-being.

Take the time to acknowledge and appreciate the progress you've made along the way, regardless of its magnitude. Embrace the journey, understanding that each day presents opportunities for growth and self-improvement. You're on the path towards becoming the version of yourself. That's definitely something worth celebrating.

Importantly, be kind and patient with yourself throughout this process. Remember that achieving health and longevity doesn't happen overnight; it's a journey. Embrace every step along the way and celebrate your accomplishments. Learn from any setbacks you encounter. Believe in your ability to make changes in your life, never losing sight of the potential that resides within you.

As we come to the end of this journey, I have full confidence that you now possess the knowledge, tools, and motivation needed to embark on your own personal quest for optimal health and longevity. Embrace this understanding and apply it to your life. Witness firsthand the impact it will have on your overall well-being.

### Here's to a life filled with vitality, joy, and longevity.

May you flourish in all aspects of your life. Serve as a source of inspiration for others. Always remember that you can shape your future. Embrace it with unwavering determination, and may your journey be marked by well-being, joy, and a long life.

# About The Author

Marta Sellers is a fresh and invigorating voice in the world of health and wellness literature. With her debut book, *"Lower Cholesterol And Triglycerides: The Ultimate Guide To Optimal Health: Transforming Your Lifestyle For Longevity,"* she brings a unique and holistic approach to tackling some of today's most prevalent health concerns.

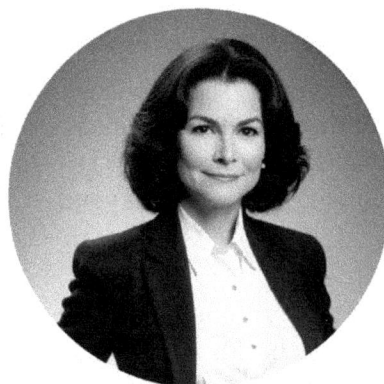

MARTA SELLERS

Marta's journey into health advocacy began with her own personal battle with high cholesterol and triglycerides, which she managed to overcome through comprehensive lifestyle changes. Her experience sparked a deep interest in holistic health, leading her to pursue studies in nutrition, exercise science, and wellness coaching.

Armed with a wealth of knowledge and a passion for helping others, Marta has worked as a wellness coach for over a decade, guiding individuals from all walks of life on their paths to better health. Her approach is not just about diet and exercise; it encompasses mental and emotional well-being, a testament to her belief in the interconnectivity of all aspects of health.

Marta's writing is characterized by its accessible and empathetic tone, making complex health topics understandable and relatable to a wide audience. In "Lower Cholesterol And Triglycerides," she combines scientific research with practical advice, drawing on both her professional expertise and personal experiences.

Beyond her writing, Marta is an avid speaker and advocate for holistic health. She regularly conducts workshops and seminars, sharing her knowledge and inspiring others to take control of their health.

Marta Sellers resides in New England, where she enjoys hiking, practicing yoga, and cooking nutritious meals. She continues to be an active member of the wellness community, constantly exploring new ways to promote holistic health and longevity.

*"Lower Cholesterol And Triglycerides: The Ultimate Guide To Optimal Health: Transforming Your Lifestyle For Longevity"* is more than a book; it's a reflection of Marta's dedication to empowering others to lead healthier, happier lives.

# More Publications From Prose Books

**No. 23-1065    1200-Calorie Diet For Senior Women:** Lose Weight, Improve Your Health, And Live Longer With a 1200-Calorie Meal Plan Daily

**No. 23-1082    Celiac Disease Cookbook For The Newly Diagnosed:** Guide To Cooking Easy And Delicious Gluten-Free Recipes For Everyone With Celiac Disease

**No. 23-1078    Fasting Your Way to Better Blood Sugar:** The Ultimate Blueprint For Effortless Weight Management And Insulin Resistance With Intermittent Fasting And Zero Sugar Diet For Diabetes Patients

No. 23-1076    Fatty Liver Diet Cookbook For Seniors Over 50: Fatty Liver Diet Cookbook For Seniors Over 50

**No 23-1079    Intermittent Fasting For Seniors:** A Beginner's Guide To Losing 10 to 30 Pounds For Senior Men And Women In 3 months. Healthy Recipes Tailored With All Diets During Your Fasting

**No. 23-1075    Intermittent Fasting For Women With PCOS:** The Science-Based Guide for Using Intermittent Fasting to Conquer PCOS, diabetes, prediabetes, Lose Weight, Balance Hormones, Increase Energy, and more

**No. 23-1071    Low Histamine Diet Cookbook And Meal Plan:** Hope and Healing In Your Kitchen: Gluten-Free and Anti-Inflammatory Recipes For Histamine Intolerance

**No. 23-1070    Ninja Speedi Keto Cookbook:** Lightning Quick Keto Meals for Busy Lives - Make the Most of Your Ninja Speedi with These Fuss-Free Keto Recipes

**No. 23-1069    Ninja Speedi Keto Cookbook:** From Fridge to Table in a Flash - 150+ Quick and Delicious Recipes for Your Ninja Speedi

**No. 23-1074    Osteoporosis Diet Cookbook For Men:** The Complete Guide to Preventing and Reversing Bone Loss with Delicious and Nutritious Recipes

**No. 23-1073    Osteoporosis Diet Cookbook Recipes For Seniors:** Delicious and Nutritious Science-Based and Calcium Fortified Recipes for Men and Women with Osteoporosis

**No. 23-1080    Plant-Based Kidney Disease Diet Cookbook For Beginners:** Beginner Friendly Low-Sodium Recipes And Guides To Prevent And Manage Chronic Kidney Disease (CKD) And Avoid Dialysis

**No. 23-1081    Pritikin Diet For Seniors:** The Complete Guide To Weight Loss And Improved Health For Seniors

**No. 23-1066    Vegan Diabetic Renal Diet Cookbook:** 125+ Delicious And Nutritious Low Sodium And Low Potassium Recipes To Help You Manage Your Diabetes And Cure Kidney Disease

**No. 23-1077    Vegan Diabetic Renal Diet Cookbook (2nd Edition):** 125+ Delicious And Nutritious Low Sodium And Low Potassium Recipes To Help You Manage Your Diabetes And Cure Kidney Disease

**Start Reading**

Scan the above code to see all the books and more…

https://prosebooks.us/books

# Thank You

Dear Readers,

As I sit down to pen this letter of gratitude, my heart is filled with an overwhelming sense of appreciation and connection. "Lower Cholesterol And Triglycerides: The Ultimate Guide To Optimal Health: Transforming Your Lifestyle For Longevity" is not just a book; it is a labor of love, a culmination of years of learning, personal experience, and the desire to make a meaningful difference in the lives of others. Your decision to embark on this journey with me is a trust I deeply cherish and value.

I am immensely grateful to each one of you who has taken the time to explore the pages of this book. Whether you are someone battling with cholesterol and triglyceride issues, a loved one supporting someone on their health journey, or simply a seeker of a healthier lifestyle, your engagement and feedback have been the driving force behind my work. This book is as much yours as it is mine, for it is your stories, challenges, and triumphs that have shaped its essence.

A special note of thanks goes to my family, friends, and colleagues, who have been unwavering in their support and encouragement. To the editorial team, healthcare professionals, and wellness advocates who have contributed their expertise and insights, your collaboration has been invaluable. Above all, I am thankful for the opportunity to share my knowledge and experiences, hoping to inspire and guide you towards a path of better health and longevity.

With heartfelt thanks,

Marta Sellers

To join our Newsletter and receive advance notification of new publications, subscribe to the Newsletter for FREE today at:

www.prosebooks.us/subscribe

www.ingramcontent.com/pod-product-compliance
Lightning Source LLC
Chambersburg PA
CBHW081551040426
42448CB00016B/3284